Everything you are abo...

- The plateau effect and plateau-breaking strategies ....
- The worst way to start ....
- Thermogenic foods 9-10
- Foods with "negative calories" 11-12
- Avoid mixing carbohydrate sources 13-14
- Hibiscus tea - a powerful secret 15-16
- Protein consumption 17-18
- The power of intermittent fasting 19-20
- Avoid liquid meals 21-22
- Yohimbine extract 23-24
- Whey protein 25-26
- Chromium & Zinc 27-28
- How to train with weights 29-30
- Peruvian Maca root 31-32
- Complex B vitamins 33-34
- Advanced training strategy 1 35-36
- Fiber in your meals 37-38
- Benefits of black tea 39-40
- Low carb high protein recipe idea 41-42
- Establish a regular eating pattern 43-44
- Creatine benefits 45-46
- Mini-Bulking strategy 47-48
- Calcium supplementation 49-50
- HIIT - Advanced fat loss strategy 51-52

	Benefits of Omega 3	53-54
	Reducing waist volume	55-56
	Fix your sleep routine	57-58
	The impact of leg training	59-60
	Accelerate your results with caffeine	61-62
	Advanced training strategy 2	63-64
	Green Tea	65-66
	Eliminating water retention	67-68
	Forskolin Extract	69-70
	Recipe idea - Protein dessert	71-72
	Chitosan for appetite reduction	73-74
	Ketogenic diet and fat consumption	75-76
	Boost your results with Ephedrine	77-78
	Advanced training strategy 3	79-80
	Recipe idea - High protein lunch	81-82
	Safflower oil	83-84
	L-carnitine	85-86
	Coenzyme Q10	87-88
	Moro orange extract	98-90
	Adequate hydration	91-92
	Psylium	93-94
	How to eliminate fecal impaction	95-96
	Recipe idea - Low carb dinner	97-100
	Selenium deficiency	101-102
	Also bet on Glucomannan	103 - 104
	Pure strength workouts	105-106
	Combine strategies intelligently	107-108

The great truth about losing weight and gaining muscle mass

What you are about to discover

When it comes to getting in shape and improving the quality of life through physical fitness, most people do not achieve solid and lasting results because they do not seek to equip themselves with the correct strategies.

And yes, it doesn't matter if your goal is muscle gain or weight control, all processes of change in our physique must be purely strategic, and implemented in an intelligent way.

There are multiple variables for us to implement in order to, together, obtain satisfactory results without unnecessary suffering and without resorting to drastic diets and methods.

- **Food planning:** The correct way to structure a diet adapted to your objective

- **Training tips:** Validated and effective strategies for optimizing an exercise routine

- **Natural extracts:** Which compounds can help you and how to implement them

- **Diet models and examples:** Which diet models can bring effective results

- **Food supplements:** Which of these can be powerful allies for fat loss and muscle gain

- **Powerful everyday boosters:** Discover specific foods with interesting properties

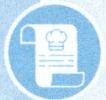

- **Homemade recipes:** Fitness recipes that will really help you stay focused on your diet

Do you know what a plateau is?

what you need to understand before starting

This is where almost 100% of people start their projects by making the main and most irreversible mistake.

Whether your goal is muscle gain or lose weight, you need to understand the logic behind your body's biological processes to obtain solid, effective results in the long term.

Before starting your project and going in search of your ideal physique, you need to equip yourself with some "plateau breaking strategies".

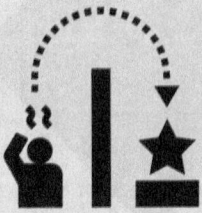

A plateau is a stage of metabolic stagnation, where you apply a very aggressive stimulus in the initial stage of your journey, and your metabolism ends up "adapting" to that radical condition.

As a direct result, this person may lose a few pounds in the short term, but will not be able to maintain this fat loss for a long time. Furthermore, this person will be left with no other resources to use and continue to lose much more weight.

Always remember: your body needs increasingly stronger stimuli to continue performing. All stimuli must be carefully dosed, and this process must be slow and gradual.

Do you know someone who started a crazy or extreme diet, hoping to lose weight quickly and ended up not being able to maintain it for many days?

tip n° 1
The plateau effect and plateau-breaking strategies

For both fat loss and muscle gain, the first and best step is to understand the nature of the plateau effect in your body.

The plateau effect in fat loss or muscle gain occurs when your progress levels off despite continued efforts.
In other words: you need to adapt your strategies before your metabolism adapts to the stimuli.

Imagine you're climbing a mountain. At first, the path is steep, and you're making quick progress. But as you ascend higher, the slope starts to level out, and you reach a plateau where the ground becomes flat.
Similarly, in your fitness journey, when you start losing fat or gaining muscle, you may see significant progress initially. However, over time, your body adapts to your exercise and diet routines, and your progress slows down, reaching a point where it seems like you're stuck on a plateau.

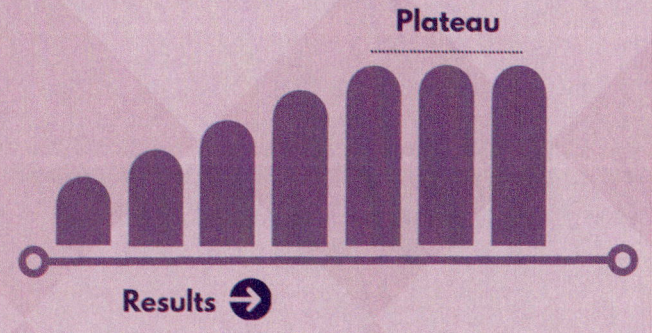

Due to our metabolism's natural ability to adapt to stimuli, all processes that seek to change our physical conditions must be implemented gradually, intelligently and in a measured manner.
A strong stimulus in the initial phase of your project will leave you without resources to continue promoting improvements in the long term and you will come across a plateau right from the start.

Fortunately, there are some important variables so that we can apply changes and promote changes at a constant pace. Imagine an airplane dashboard with several buttons:

- Diet and calorie consumption;
- Exercise intensity;
- Changes in eating patterns;
- Advanced workout strategies;
- Implementation of some compounds and food supplements;
- Some other interesting plateau breaking strategies;

Now that you understand the main biological mechanism of our body when we try to implement drastic changes, you are able to start implementing some of these strategies and achieve constant and satisfactory results by gradually applying effective stimulus.

From this perspective, we recommend that you adapt some of these important tips little by little. And each time the results appear to slow down or stop, you can implement another strategy or increase the intensity so that you always continue to make progress.

tip n° 2
Restrictive diets: The worst way to start

According to the logic of the plateau effect, when we talk about gaining muscle mass or losing fat, the general idea is that your body does not want drastic changes and will always try to adapt to the stimuli applied.

Suppose your goal is to lose weight. You are excited about a diet model you read about. In this diet you will restrict your meals to just salad and protein sources, making your caloric consumption practically zero directly on the day you decide to embark on this diet.

It may seem like a great idea at first, and you may even lose some weight in the first few days of following this strict diet.
However, you still don't know but your process is already doomed to failure at this stage. Starting an extremely restrictive diet has two devastating consequences:

- The first of them is that even if we persists for several months in this eating model, we won't be able to lose much more than a few pounds, and will be stuck in a large stage of stagnation despite the calorie intake being at zero. Yes, this is possible, as your body can be smarter than you and adapt to this condition.

- The second consequence is that it will be extremely difficult and painful to maintain such a low calorie level for a long time. It is common for some people to go back to binge eating, even gaining more weight than before.

The correct way to start and progress with a diet

An effective and intelligent diet must be implemented progressively. Whether your goal is to lose weight or gain muscle mass (it is possible to do both simultaneously).

1. Establish a standard diet that you feel comfortable and satisfied with, without feeling hungry during the day.

2. Get into the habit of weighing the "macronutrients" or meal portion volumes to make it easier to control, monitor your caloric intake and progress gradually.

3. In this first approach, the most important "macronutrient" will be carbohydrate sources, as they are the most responsible for your total caloric intake.

4. Starting from your initially established standard meal, try to reduce the amounts of carbohydrate sources periodically (weekly or monthly) by making subtle adjustments so that your diet remains comfortable but guarantees a small caloric cut.

5. You can replace the amounts of carbohydrates subtracted with sources of protein or fiber (we will talk about other details later).

6. As you progress, try to replace your carbohydrate sources with higher glycemic indices (pasta, rice, white bread) with others with lower glycemic indices (Whole Grain Bread, Brown Rice, Quinoa, Sweet Potatoes, etc).

tip nº 3 — Implement some thermogenic foods

Some foods and natural extracts have the interesting property of "accelerating" the human metabolism, making them potential allies for weight loss.

These are commonly called "natural thermogenics" and have some compounds that literally act as catalysts for some processes in the body, giving a "Boost" in biochemical reactions.

Some of these biochemical reactions literally involve an increase in body temperature, dilation of blood vessels and increased blood flow.

In addition to promoting a considerable increase in caloric consumption, these foods are also related to reducing appetite and hunger as they normally also contain phytocompounds capable of acting as adrenergic stimulants.

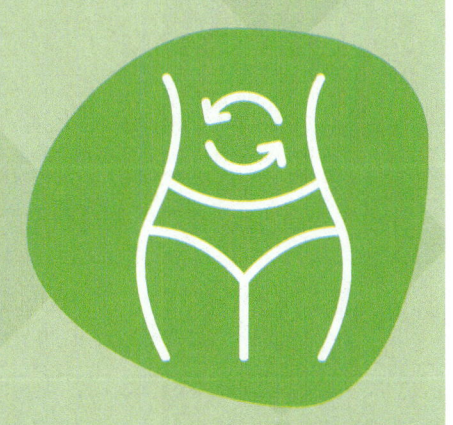

This occurs because the compounds present in these foods increase the secretion of serotonin by neuronal cells in the intestine in response to intestinal stimuli, which supposedly reduces food intake; and would reduce the secretion of ghrelin, a hormone that stimulates appetite and food intake, by gastric cells.

Some common examples of natural thermogenics

Ginger: Ginger has thermogenic properties that can help increase metabolism and promote fat burning.

Cinnamon: Cinnamon may help regulate blood sugar levels and improve insulin sensitivity, which can indirectly support weight loss efforts.

Turmeric: Curcumin, the active compound in turmeric, has been shown to have thermogenic properties and may help increase metabolism.

Chili Peppers: Capsaicin, the compound responsible for the spicy heat in chili peppers, can boost metabolism and increase the body's calorie-burning process.

Coconut Oil: Medium-chain triglycerides (MCTs) found in coconut oil have been shown to increase metabolism and promote fat burning.

Apple Cider Vinegar: Some studies suggest that consuming apple cider vinegar may help increase metabolism and promote fat loss, although more research is needed.

Garlic: Garlic contains allicin, a compound that may help boost metabolism and promote fat burning.

These resources are an excellent tip to further boost your results. However, just consuming these foods cannot guarantee effective weight loss, as it is essential that your metabolism is in a calorie deficit (Spending more calories than we consume).

tip n° 4
Try foods with "negative calories"

Yes, you read that right. What if I told you that there is a class of foods that you can consume in any quantity and without feeling guilty.

In fact, what if I told you that it was even possible to burn calories simply by eating? Seems like a lie, right? But this category of food exists and can be a great strategic ally to reduce hunger or binge eating and assist in your weight control process.

In reality, all foods have a caloric value, however some of these foods have an extremely fibrous or protein composition, making them difficult to digest and process by the body.

As a direct consequence, our body ends up releasing a lot of energy consuming these foods, making the total caloric balance "negative". It's as if our body did a gym session to process this meal.

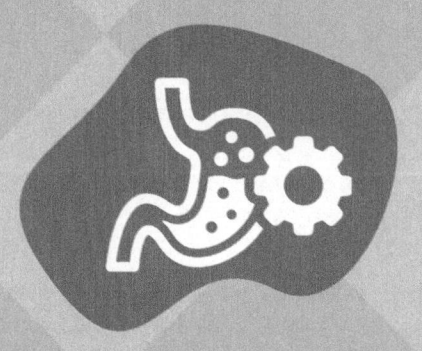

And spending calories eating is a brilliant idea considering that we want to lose fat without feeling hungry, do you agree?

Some of these foods with negative caloric loads are:

Whole Grains: Whole grains like oats, quinoa, and brown rice require more energy to digest compared to refined grains, leading to increased calorie burning.

Lean Protein: Foods high in protein, such as chicken breast, turkey, fish, and tofu, require more energy to digest and metabolize, leading to a higher metabolic rate.

Leafy Greens: Vegetables like spinach, kale, and Swiss chard are low in calories and rich in fiber, vitamins, and minerals, supporting overall health and weight management.

Watermelon: Watermelon is an excellent ally for weight loss as its composition is almost exclusively fiber and water.

Eggs: Eggs are a great source of high-quality protein and contain nutrients like vitamin D and choline, which can support metabolism and fat burning.

Almonds: Almonds are rich in protein, healthy fats, and fiber, all of which can help increase metabolism and promote feelings of fullness.

Yogurt: Yogurt, especially Greek yogurt, is high in protein and can help increase metabolism and promote fat loss when consumed as part of a balanced diet.

Brazil Nuts: Brazil nuts are a good source of selenium, a mineral that supports thyroid function and metabolism.

tip n° 5
Avoid mixing carbohydrate sources

This is a tip that can optimize your fat loss process or prevent the gain of abdominal fat for those who want to keep their fat percentage low.

What is glycemic index?

Imagine you're eating a slice of bread. After you eat it, your body breaks down the carbohydrates in that bread into sugar, which then enters your bloodstream. **The glycemic index (GI)** is a way to measure how quickly that sugar from the bread enters your bloodstream.

High GI
- White Bread
- White Rice
- Sugary Cereals
- Pasta

Low GI
- Sweet Potatoes
- Oatmeal
- Lentils
- Chickpeas

Foods with a high GI make your blood sugar rise quickly because they're broken down fast, like sugary snacks. Foods with a low GI release sugar more slowly into your bloodstream, like whole grains and vegetables.

So, the GI helps you understand how different foods affect your blood sugar levels. If you're trying to manage your blood sugar, choosing foods with a lower GI can help keep your levels more stable.

Carbohydrate mix

Here there are two pieces of information you need to understand about the glycemic index of foods:

1 **Whenever possible, choose carbohydrates with low glycemic indices as high glycemic index foods can contribute to weight gain because they cause rapid spikes in blood sugar, leading to increased insulin production and potential storage of excess calories as fat.**

2 **Mixing different carbohydrates in the same meal can potentially contribute to weight gain because it can lead to a higher overall glycemic load, causing more significant spikes in blood sugar levels and increased insulin secretion, which may promote fat storage over time.**

This rapid rise in blood sugar triggers your body to release insulin to help regulate it. Insulin's main job is to shuttle glucose (sugar) from your bloodstream into your cells for energy or storage. However, when there's an excess of glucose and insulin in your bloodstream, your body may prioritize **storing that excess energy as fat.**

In conclusion, if you limit yourself to consuming a single source of carbohydrate per meal, you will certainly be avoiding a rapid accumulation of fat, especially visceral and abdominal fat.

tip nº 6
Hibiscus tea a powerful secret

Hibiscus is a reddish flower, most common in tropical regions. The flower has several medicinal and culinary applications and is proven to be a powerful weight loss ally, despite being little known.

The flower has phytochemical components capable of acting in multiple ways against fat gain, with direct actions ranging from appetite suppression to fat metabolism. For this reason, Hibiscus deserves this important position in this material.

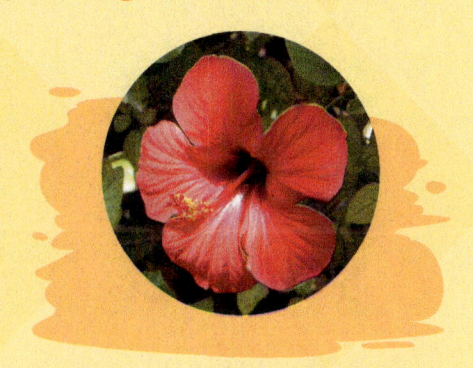

- **Metabolism Boosting:** Some studies suggest that hibiscus tea may have the ability to boost metabolism. An increased metabolic rate can help the body burn fat more efficiently, contributing to weight loss.

- **Appetite Suppressant:** Hibiscus tea contains several compounds that might influence appetite control, but the most noted one is hydroxycitric acid (HCA), which can help reduce overall calorie intake.

- **Diuretic Properties:** Hibiscus is known for its diuretic effect. This property helps rid the body of excess water weight and sodium, reducing bloating and minor swelling.

Effect on Cholesterol and Lipid Levels:
Hibiscus tea has been studied for its impact on cholesterol levels. Some research indicates that it can lower total cholesterol, low-density lipoprotein (LDL) cholesterol, and triglycerides while increasing (HDL) cholesterol. Improving these markers can help with weight management and prevent further complications linked with obesity.

Digestive Aid: Hibiscus tea is sometimes credited with helping to improve digestion. It can help to regularize bowel movements and improve gut health, which is important for weight loss and overall wellness.

Here's how you can prepare it in just a few steps:

1. **Measure the Hibiscus**: Typically, use about 1 to 2 teaspoons of dried hibiscus flowers per cup of water, depending on how strong you like your tea.

2. **Steep the Hibiscus:** Add the dried hibiscus flowers to the boiling water. Remove from heat and let them steep for about 5 to 10 minutes. The longer you steep, the deeper the flavor and color.

3. **Strain the Tea**: Use a fine mesh strainer to remove the flowers from the water. Dispose of the used hibiscus flowers.

tip n° 7
Increase protein consumption

Maintaining a high protein intake has enormous benefits both for fat loss and for gaining and maintaining lean mass.
Let's talk about the main ones and also the ideal amount of protein portions that you should already be implementing into your eating routine to significantly improve your body composition.

Increases Muscle Mass and Strength:
As you may already know, the greater your muscle mass, the faster your basal metabolism, and this means that you can also lose fat more quickly and efficiently.
And in this mechanism, proteins are the main "raw materials" essential for muscle synthesis.

Boosts Metabolism: High protein intake can increase the rate at which your body burns calories by boosting your metabolic rate. This happens through the thermic effect of food, as protein requires more energy to digest compared to fats and carbohydrates.

Reduces Appetite and Hunger Levels / Curbs cravings:
Protein is **3 times more satiating** than carbohydrates or fats. It helps you feel fuller for longer, reducing the need to snack between meals and decreasing overall calorie intake.
Studies have shown that eating a high-protein diet can help in reducing cravings and the desire for late-night snacking.

What is the ideal portion of protein I should eat daily?

Fortunately, there is a very simple calculation that we can do to find out what amount of protein is ideal and adapted for each person.

For People Who Do Not Train (Sedentary Individuals):

- The recommended daily intake of protein for sedentary individuals is around <u>0.8 grams</u> per kilogram of body weight.
- For example, if someone weighs 70 kilograms (about 154 pounds), they would aim for approximately 56 grams of protein per day.

For People Who Workout (Active Individuals):

- Active individuals, especially those engaging in strength training or endurance exercise, may require more protein to support muscle repair and growth.
- The general guideline for active individuals is to consume between <u>1.2 to 2.2 grams</u> of protein per kilogram of body weight.
- For someone weighing 70 kilograms, this would mean consuming between 84 to 154 grams of protein per day, depending on the intensity and duration of their workouts.

These calculations are an estimate that can help us find our ideal goal for daily protein consumption.
You won't need to meticulously calculate the protein content of each food. Overall this calculation gives us a good starting point.

tip n° 8
The power of intermittent fasting

If you don't already know, intermittent fasting is an excellent ace up your sleeve to break a plateau and overcome a stage of stagnation in results. Intermittent fasting directly affects your insulin resistance, which can benefit both fat loss and lean mass gain.

If you are trying to lose weight and are continually reducing your daily calories and gradually increasing your exercise routine and still feel like you are no longer losing weight, try a few weeks of intermittent fasting. This powerful strategy can move things forward.

If you are on a diet focused on gaining muscle mass, intermittent fasting for a short period of time can also help you change your insulin resistance, which can be beneficial for muscle gain as well.

Think of intermittent fasting as giving your body a break from eating for a certain period of time, then eating during a specific window. Here's how it works:

1. **Fasting Period**: This is when you don't eat anything for a set amount of time. It could be overnight while you sleep or for several hours during the day.
2. **Eating Window**: This is the time when you're allowed to eat. It might be a few hours or up to eight hours, depending on the fasting plan you're following.

So, for example, if you're doing a 16/8 intermittent fasting plan:

- You might fast for 16 hours (including the time you're sleeping).
- Then, you have an 8-hour window where you can eat your meals and snacks for the day.

The idea is that by giving your body this fasting period, you're helping it burn fat more efficiently and reap other health benefits like improved brain function and better blood sugar control.
It's important to find a fasting schedule that works for you and fits into your lifestyle. And remember, always listen to your body.

The benefits of intermittent fasting extend beyond just aesthetic benefits:

Brain Boost: Some studies suggest intermittent fasting may enhance cognitive function, focus, and protect against age-related brain diseases like Alzheimer's.

Energy Enhancer: By giving your digestive system a break, intermittent fasting frees up energy, reducing feelings of sluggishness and helping you power through your day.

Blood Sugar Stabilizer: Intermittent fasting can regulate blood sugar levels, improving insulin sensitivity and lowering the risk of type 2 diabetes.

Heart Health: Intermittent fasting is linked to improvements in heart health, including lower blood pressure, cholesterol levels, and inflammation markers, supporting overall cardiovascular well-being.

tip n° 9 Avoid liquid meals

In the previous chapter we discussed a great alternative to reducing your insulin resistance, which is an excellent thing, for better health in general or for aesthetic purposes such as fat loss and mass gain. However, now let's talk about a great enemy of weight loss. Liquid meals high in sugar may be greatly increasing your insulin resistance and preventing you from achieving your results.

Liquid meals, such as shakes, smoothies, and even natural fruit juices can seem like a convenient option for weight loss, but there are a few reasons why they may not be the best choice:

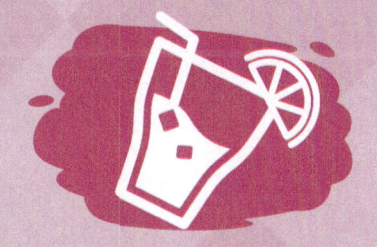

- **Faster Digestion:** When you drink a meal, it doesn't take as long to digest as when you eat solid foods. This means the calories from liquid meals can be absorbed more quickly into your bloodstream, potentially leading to a spike in blood sugar levels.

- **Less Satiety:** Unlike solid foods that require chewing and take up space in your stomach, liquid meals may not make you feel as full or satisfied. This can lead to consuming more calories overall throughout the day, which can contribute to weight gain.

Most people don't know this, but even fresh juices or fruit shakes can pose a threat to your weight loss progress.

To <u>reduce the glycemic index</u> of a liquid meal and help stabilize blood sugar levels, you can add ingredients that are lower in carbohydrates and higher in fiber, protein, and healthy fats. Here are some options:

Leafy Greens: Add spinach, kale, or other leafy greens to your smoothie. They're high in fiber, which can help slow down the absorption of sugar into the bloodstream.

Low-Glycemic Fruits: Choose fruits that have a lower glycemic index, such as berries (like strawberries, blueberries, and raspberries), cherries, or apples. These fruits contain less sugar and more fiber compared to high-glycemic fruits like bananas or mangoes.

Healthy Fats: Include sources of healthy fats such as avocado, nut butter, or coconut milk in your smoothie. Fats can help slow down the digestion of carbohydrates, resulting in a lower glycemic response.

Protein: Add protein-rich ingredients like Greek yogurt, silken tofu, or protein powder to your liquid meal.

Fiber-Rich Seeds: Incorporate chia seeds, flaxseeds, or hemp seeds into your smoothie for an extra boost of fiber. These seeds also provide healthy fats and protein.

Spices: Sprinkle in cinnamon, ginger, or turmeric to add flavor to your liquid meal while also potentially helping to stabilize blood sugar levels.

tip n° 10
Yohimbine extract a little explored ally

Yohimbine, extracted from the bark of the yohimbe tree, is a natural supplement renowned for its ability to increase energy levels, promote fat loss, and improve libido, making it a great addition to your fa

There is a specific type of abdominal fat that you will hardly be able to lose, even with great effort, physical activity and strict diets. We are talking about visceral fat.

Yohimbine has been studied for its potential to target stubborn fat, including visceral fat. One way yohimbine may help reduce visceral fat is by stimulating the release of adrenaline, which can increase the breakdown of fat stored in fat cells. Additionally, yohimbine may block certain receptors in fat cells, preventing them from holding on to fat.

The use of yohimbine extract is recommended in the more advanced phases of your project, as its main benefit is to reduce the fat that we cannot eliminate through other stimuli.

The effects of yohimbine extract are similar to those of caffeine, acting as a powerful natural thermogenic, accelerating metabolic reactions, and may slightly increase body temperature as a result.

The main studied benefits of yohimbine extract

Fat Burning: Yohimbine may aid in fat loss by increasing the breakdown of stored fat, particularly stubborn fat areas.

Energy Boost: It can provide a natural energy boost by stimulating the release of adrenaline, helping you feel more energized.

Appetite Suppression: Yohimbine may help reduce appetite and cravings, making it easier to stick to a calorie-controlled diet.

Improved Circulation: Yohimbine has vasodilatory effects, which means it can widen blood vessels and improve blood flow, potentially benefiting conditions like erectile dysfunction.

Enhanced Athletic Performance: Some research suggests that yohimbine may improve athletic performance by increasing endurance and reducing fatigue.

Dosage and how to use yohimbine

Start Low, Go Slow: Begin with a low dose of yohimbine, typically around 5-10 milligrams per day, to assess tolerance and minimize potential side effects.

Timing Matters: Take yohimbine on an empty stomach, preferably in the morning or before exercise, to maximize its fat-burning and energy-boosting effects.

Gradual Increase: If tolerated well, gradually increase the dose up to 20-30 milligrams per day, divided into two or three doses, to further enhance its benefits.

tip n° 11
Whey protein

Whey protein is isolated milk protein. It is one of the most interesting alternatives to increase your daily protein portion as milk protein has a very high biological value. This means that practically 100% of whey protein can be absorbed by our body, unlike other sources of protein, such as soy, where only 70% is actually assimilated by the body.

Whey protein is highly recommended for people of all ages and conditions. Regardless of whether your goal is to gain muscle mass, lose fat or both. As previously mentioned in the chapter dedicated to proteins, you can use whey protein to balance the consumption of proteins in your meals.

It is possible that some people find it difficult to consume large portions of other sources of protein, such as meat and eggs, to maintain a recommended daily protein intake.
In this scenario, whey protein comes in as the best alternative.

- **Boosts Metabolism:** Whey protein can help increase your metabolism, which means you burn more calories throughout the day, even when you're at rest.
- **Enhances Muscle Growth:** Packed with essential amino acids, whey protein is great for muscle repair and growth after workouts, helping you build lean muscle mass.
- **Reduces Hunger:** Whey protein is quite filling, which can help curb your appetite and reduce cravings, making it easier to stick to a healthy diet.

It is important to note that you can choose to drink your protein shake pure (with water only) or add a source of fiber to the drink depending on your goals or whichever is more comfortable for your digestion.

Pure Whey Protein: Drinking whey protein on its own is fantastic for a quick absorption of protein, ideal for post-workout recovery when your body needs protein fast to repair and build muscle.

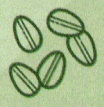

Whey Protein with fiber sources: Mixing oats or other fiber sources with your whey protein provides a more balanced shake. This is a great idea to make the protein release more slowly, which can be beneficial for sustained energy and satiety. It's a good choice for a meal replacement or a hearty breakfast. Adding a fiber source (like psyllium husk, chia seeds, or flaxseeds) to whey protein can enhance digestive health and help keep you feeling full longer. This option might appeal to those looking to lose weight or improve digestive function.

The best option depends on what you need nutritionally. For quick muscle recovery, go with pure whey protein post-workout. For a meal replacement or if you need more energy and satiety, adding oats or fiber can be beneficial.

tip n° 12
Add Chromium & Zinc in your diet

Maintaining a balanced diet, consuming adequate doses of all essential minerals, although highly recommended, cannot actively contribute to weight loss. However, a nutritional deficiency in some minerals may be a factor preventing you from losing weight.

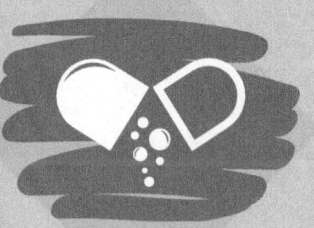

The minerals Zinc and Chromium are the mineral components proven to be directly active in the fat metabolism process. They play an extremely important role in hormonal and insulin regulation.

Zinc and chromium deficiencies can hinder weight loss by disrupting metabolic processes related to glucose regulation, appetite control, and energy metabolism, which are essential for efficient fat burning and maintaining a healthy weight.

If you are on a calorie restricted diet and are trying to lose weight and are finding it difficult to make progress, try checking the mineral dosages in your diet.

A poor diet, without vegetables, greens, and little diversity can be alarming for a lack of minerals, and some of these interesting nutrients are a little more difficult to obtain through the diet.

Important sources of Zinc:

- Oysters and Shellfish (such as crab, lobster, and shrimp)
- Chicken, pork, turkey and beef
- Legumes (such as lentils, chickpeas, and beans)
- Nuts and seeds (such as pumpkin seeds, cashews, and almonds)
- Whole grains (such as wheat germ and quinoa)
- Dairy products (such as milk, cheese, and yogurt)

Important sources of Chromium:

- Whole grains (such as whole wheat bread, oats, and barley)
- Green beans, broccoli, Asparagus, Spinach
- Nuts and seeds (Brazil nuts, peanuts, and sunflower seeds)
- Meat (such as beef and chicken)
- Seafood (such as clams and mussels)
- Mushrooms

If you are unsure about the nutritional value of your daily diet, try supplementing with these minerals.

Recommended daily allowances

Zinc :
- Adult men: 11 milligrams
- Adult women: 8 milligrams
- Pregnant women may need slightly more.

Chromium :
- Adult men: 35 micrograms
- Adult women: 25 micrograms
- Pregnant women may also need slightly more.

tip n° 13
The correct way to train with weights

If your goal is to lose fat you need to understand that increasing your muscle mass is the most impactful thing you can do to accelerate your results.
This happens because the more developed your muscle mass is, the faster your basal metabolism is, and your body will be able to metabolize fats at a much faster rate.

And if your goal is to gain muscle mass, we don't even need to comment on how necessary weight exercises are. You will now understand all the types of weight training and how to perform them correctly depending on your objective.

Let's break down the three types of weight workouts

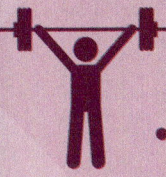

Strength Training

- Goal: To increase overall strength, allowing you to lift heavier weights.

- How to Do It: Focus on heavy weights with low repetitions. Typically, you do 1 to 6 repetitions per set with longer rest periods (2 to 5 minutes) between sets. Compound exercises like squats, deadlifts, and bench presses are commonly used.

- Example Workout: Do 4 sets of 5 repetitions of deadlifts, with a 3-minute rest between each set.

Resistance Training (Endurance)

- Goal: To improve muscle endurance and cardiovascular health.

- How to Do It: Use lighter weights with higher repetitions. Aim for 12 to 20 repetitions per set, with shorter rest periods (30 seconds to 1 minute). Exercises that keep your heart rate up, like bodyweight movements, are common.

- Example Workout: Do 3 sets of 15 repetitions of push-ups, with a 30-second rest between sets.

Hypertrophy Training

- Goal: To increase muscle size and definition.

- How to Do It: Use moderate weights with moderate repetitions. Typically, you aim for 6 to 12 repetitions per set with moderate rest periods (1 to 2 minutes). Isolation exercises and a mix of compound movements are key.

- Example Workout: Do 4 sets of 10 repetitions of bicep curls, with a 1.5-minute rest between sets.

Each type of workout serves a different purpose, so choose based on your fitness goals. If you want to increase raw strength, go for strength training. If you need to improve endurance and conditioning, opt for resistance training. For muscle growth and definition, hypertrophy training will be your best bet.

tip n° 14 Try Peruvian Maca

Peruvian maca root is an exotic superfood native to the high Andes of Peru, often hailed for its energy-boosting and hormone-balancing properties. This unique root is packed with vitamins, minerals, and plant compounds that make it a fantastic addition to any fitness-focused diet.

Numerous studies indicate that the administration of Maca extract can stimulate the endogenous production of testosterone (which is beneficial in both men and women). This effect is mainly proven in people with a hormonal disorder or imbalance.

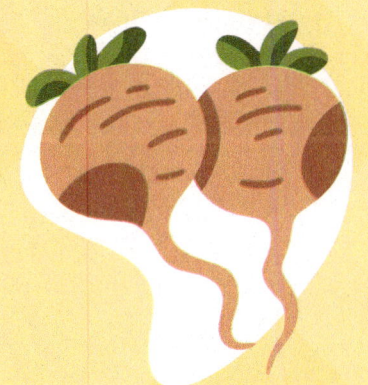

When it comes to weight loss, maca root's adaptogenic qualities help reduce stress and curb emotional eating, supporting a more balanced approach to shedding pounds. Plus, its natural energy-boosting effects can supercharge your workouts, allowing you to push harder and burn more calories! For those aiming to gain muscle, maca's ability to support hormone balance can enhance muscle growth and recovery, giving you an edge in your training regimen. So, whether you're looking to slim down or bulk up, consider studying Peruvian maca a little better and adapting it to your routine.

Main known benefits of Maca

Energy Boost: Maca root is known to increase energy and endurance, helping you power through workouts and burn more calories, which is beneficial for weight loss and muscle gain.

Improved Stamina: Maca can enhance physical stamina, allowing for longer and more intense workouts, which can contribute to muscle growth and increased calorie expenditure.

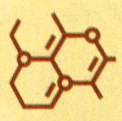

Hormone Balance: Maca may help balance hormones, which can support a healthy metabolism and reduce stress-related weight gain.

Muscle Recovery: Maca's nutrient-rich profile, including essential amino acids, can support muscle recovery and growth after exercise.

Improved Mood: Maca's mood-enhancing properties can help maintain motivation and a positive outlook, aiding in adherence to a healthy lifestyle.

Recommended daily dose

To get the most out of maca root, the ideal dosage is generally between 1,500 and 3,000 milligrams per day. You can start with a lower dose to see how your body responds, then gradually increase it if needed. It's best to divide your daily dose into two or three smaller doses throughout the day, like adding it to your morning smoothie and afternoon snack.

tip n° 15
Complex B vitamins

We talked earlier about minerals that can potentially impact your results, and it is important to note that some people are also severely deficient in vitamins, as a result of a diet that is not well balanced or is low in relevant vitamin sources.
The ideal is an adequate consumption of all vitamins and minerals, however some of these vitamins are proven to be involved in fat and muscle metabolism processes.

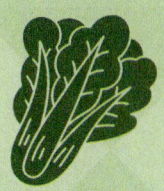

B complex vitamins play crucial roles in fat metabolism by acting as coenzymes that facilitate essential metabolic processes. For instance, vitamins B1 (thiamine) and B5 (pantothenic acid) are involved in the conversion of fats to energy through their roles in synthesizing and utilizing acetyl-CoA. Vitamin B2 (riboflavin) and B3 (niacin) help produce energy from fats by participating in the electron transport chain. B6 (pyridoxine) assists in breaking down proteins and fats, while B7 (biotin) aids in synthesizing fatty acids. Collectively, these vitamins ensure that fats are efficiently converted into energy, supporting overall metabolic health.

Most people have some degree or type of deficiency in certain nutrients, and this situation is unfortunately more common than you think. But you don't want the reason your body can't metabolize fats to be due to an easy-to-treat nutritional deficiency that prevents these reactions from happening naturally.

B complex vitamins are found in a variety of natural food sources, making it possible and easy to obtain them through a balanced diet. Here's where you can find different B vitamins:

- **Vitamin B1** (Thiamine): Whole grains, pork, seeds, and nuts.
- **Vitamin B2** (Riboflavin): Milk, cheese, eggs, leafy vegetables, liver, and kidney.
- **Vitamin B3** (Niacin): Meat, fish, wheat flour, eggs, and milk.
- **Vitamin B5** (Pantothenic Acid): Chicken, beef, potatoes, oats, cereals, liver, kidney, yeast, eggs, and dairy products.
- **Vitamin B6** (Pyridoxine): Chicken, turkey, tuna, salmon, lentils, sunflower seeds, cheese, brown rice, and carrots.
- **Vitamin B7** (Biotin): Eggs, almonds, nuts, legumes, whole grains, milk, and meats.
- **Vitamin B9** (Folate): Leafy green vegetables, legumes, seeds, liver, and certain fruits.
- **Vitamin B12** (Cobalamin): Meat, fish, dairy products, and fortified cereals.

tip n° 16
Advanced training strategy - Drop set

Now that you probably understand the importance of increasing your percentage of lean mass even to enhance your weight loss, it's time to talk about an interesting and advanced plateau-breaking strategy for your strength training.

As previously mentioned, in basic weight training for hypertrophy (increase in muscle mass) you perform repetitive movements of contracting and relaxing the muscles, limiting yourself to a number of repetitions of up to 12 times. Do you remember?

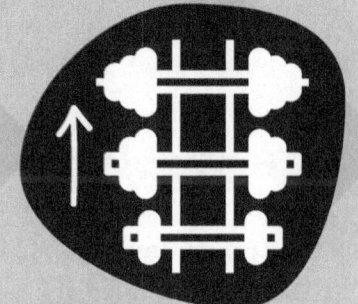

Although this strategy is a good starting point for beginners with weight training, very soon this pattern of repetitions and weights will no longer bring many results and you will stagnate on a plateau. You will need another suitable strategy to continue giving your muscles a growth stimulus.

The drop set strategy in weight training is an intense technique where you perform a set of an exercise until failure, then immediately reduce the weight and continue to lift for more reps until failure. This process can be repeated multiple times without resting between sets, significantly increasing muscle fatigue and growth by pushing muscles beyond their usual limits. Drop sets are highly effective for breaking through plateaus and maximizing muscle hypertrophy.

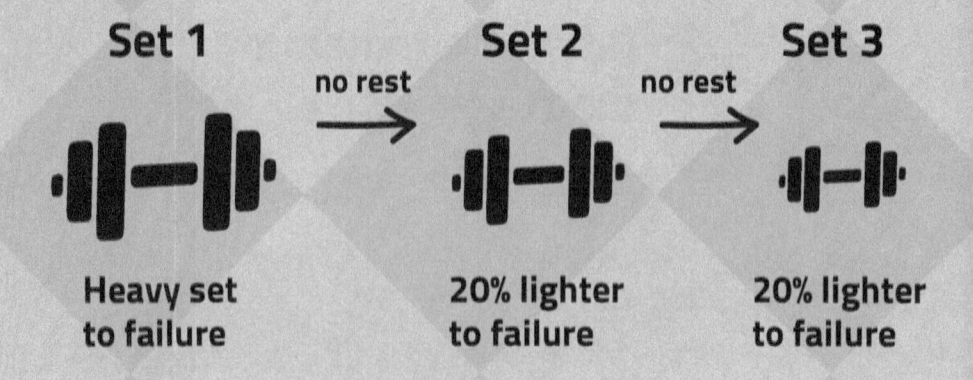

Set 1		Set 2		Set 3
🏋️	no rest →	🏋️	no rest →	🏋️
Heavy set to failure		**20% lighter to failure**		**20% lighter to failure**

1. **Initial Set:** Begin by performing bicep curls with a weight you can lift for 8-10 reps until muscle failure—meaning you can't perform another full rep with good form.
2. **First Drop:** Immediately reduce the weight by 20-30% and continue to perform more curls until failure once again.
3. **Subsequent Drops:** You can opt to reduce the weight again by a similar percentage and repeat, continuing to curl until you can no longer perform a rep due to fatigue.

This method dramatically increases the time under tension and the total volume of work performed by the muscles, both critical factors for muscle growth. By pushing the muscles past their usual limits, drop sets create significant metabolic stress—leading to <u>enhanced muscle hypertrophy and increased calorie burn</u>, as the body works harder to recover from the intense exertion. Compared to traditional training methods that involve resting between sets, drop sets maintain a higher heart rate and metabolic rate, potentially optimizing fat loss while building muscle more efficiently.

tip n° 17
Add more fiber

Dietary fibers do not have a complex nutritional value but added to your diet are extremely important components, especially for people who are looking to lose weight and control their appetite.

- **Increases Satiety:** Fiber absorbs water and expands in your stomach, making you feel full sooner and longer after meals, which helps reduce overall calorie intake.

- **Slows Digestion:** By slowing down the digestion process, fiber helps maintain steady blood sugar levels, preventing energy crashes and reducing hunger pangs.

- **Low in Calories:** High-fiber foods tend to be lower in calories relative to their volume, allowing you to eat larger portions without packing on extra calories.

- **Boosts Metabolism:** Some types of fiber, like those found in whole grains, can slightly increase your metabolic rate by requiring more energy to break down.

- **Improves Gut Health:** Fiber promotes a healthy digestive system by supporting beneficial gut bacteria, which play a role in weight management and metabolic health.

Adding more fiber to your daily meals is easier than you might think! Start by swapping out white breads, pastas, and rice for their whole grain counterparts—it's a simple switch that packs a fibrous punch. Incorporate more fruits and vegetables into your meals; they're not only nutritious but also great sources of fiber. You can add berries to your morning oatmeal, munch on carrots or celery with hummus as a snack, and toss extra vegetables into soups, stews, and salads. Additionally, adding legumes like beans or lentils to dishes boosts both your protein and fiber intake.

Here are some interesting examples

- **Beans and lentils:** Great for soups, stews, and salads.
- **Whole grains:** Such as oats, quinoa, and whole wheat pasta.
- **Nuts and seeds:** Snack on them or sprinkle over salads.
- **Berries:** Strawberries, raspberries, and blackberries.
- **Apples and pears:** With the skin on for extra fiber.
- **Vegetables:** Carrots, broccoli, and leafy greens.
- **Potatoes:** Especially with the skin on.

It is worth noting that fiber does not have any caloric value, but together with your meals they have the power to reduce the caloric impact and glycemic index of your meals, preventing weight gain.

tip n° 18
Implement black tea

Here's another powerful natural extract tip to boost your metabolism promoting fat oxidation, and enhancing energy levels, making it easier to burn calories and stay active throughout the day.

Remember that we talked about compounds and foods with thermogenic properties earlier? Here is a complete combo, with thermogenic properties linked to caffeine as well as other strong antioxidant properties coming from various phytochemical compounds.

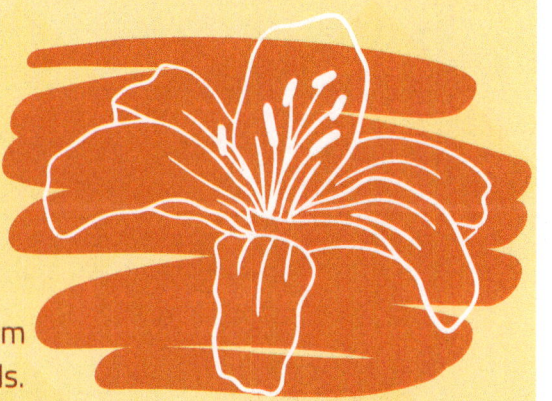

Black tea is a popular beverage made from the leaves of the Camellia sinensis plant. It's known for its robust flavor and dark color.

Let's talk about its fantastic benefits, especially for fat loss:

- **Boosts Metabolism:** Black tea contains compounds like caffeine and flavonoids that can speed up your metabolism, helping your body burn calories more efficiently.

- **Promotes Fat Oxidation:** Drinking black tea may encourage your body to break down fat stores for energy, which can support weight loss efforts.

Enhances Energy Levels: With a moderate amount of caffeine, black tea can give you a natural energy boost, helping you stay active and burn more calories throughout the day.

Reduces Hunger Cravings: Black tea's rich phytocompounds and caffeine content can help suppress appetite and reduce cravings, making it easier to stick to your weight loss goals.

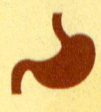

Improves Digestion: Some studies suggest that the polyphenols in black tea may support healthy digestion, which is essential for efficient nutrient absorption and overall well-being.

To prepare black tea correctly and optimize the extraction of its flavors and benefits, follow these simple steps:

1. **Boil Water:** Start by boiling fresh, filtered water. The ideal temperature for black tea is just off the boil, around 200-212°F (93-100°C).
2. **Pre-Warm the Teapot or Cup**: Swirl a little hot water in your teapot or cup, then discard.
3. **Add Tea:** Use 1 teaspoon of loose-leaf tea or 1 tea bag per cup.
4. **Pour Hot Water:** Pour over the tea leaves or tea bag, ensuring they're submerged.
5. **Steep for 3-5 Minutes:** Steep for the desired strength, then remove the tea leaves or tea bag.

tip n° 19
Low carb high protein recipe idea - Breakfast

Protein-Packed Breakfast Burrito

This breakfast burrito is high in protein, fiber, and essential nutrients, making it a great choice for fueling your day and supporting your fitness goals!

Ingredients:

- 2 large whole wheat tortillas
- 4 large eggs
- 1/4 cup diced bell peppers
- 1/4 cup diced onions
- 1/4 cup diced tomatoes
- 1/4 cup cooked black beans
- 1/4 cup shredded cheddar cheese (reduced-fat)
- Salt and pepper to taste
- Optional toppings: salsa, avocado slices, Greek yogurt

Instructions:

- In a non-stick skillet over medium heat, sauté the diced bell peppers and onions until they start to soften, about 3-4 minutes.

- Crack the eggs into the skillet with the peppers and onions. Scramble them until they're fully cooked.

- Stir in the diced tomatoes and cooked black beans. Cook for an additional minute to heat through.

- Warm the tortillas in the microwave for about 15-20 seconds to make them pliable.

- Divide the egg mixture evenly between the tortillas, placing it in the center of each one.

- Sprinkle shredded cheddar cheese over the egg mixture on each tortilla.

- Season with salt and pepper to taste. Fold the sides of each tortilla over the filling, then roll it up tightly into a burrito.

Serve immediately, with optional toppings like salsa, avocado slices, or Greek yogurt on the side.

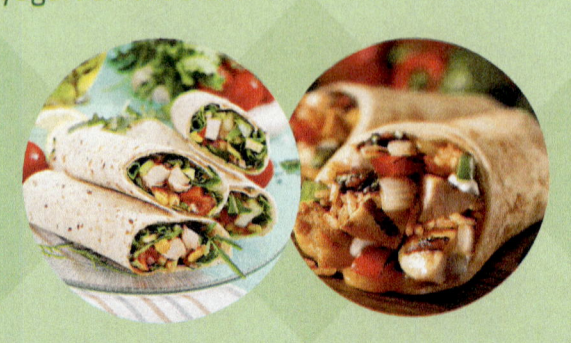

tip n° 20 Establish a regular eating pattern

A lot of people don't stick to a regular meal schedule. One day they eat breakfast, but the next day they skip it. Sometimes they have lunch at noon, but other times it's much later.

Although little known or talked about, this habit of distributing daily meals without organized patterns could be unbalancing your metabolism and sabotaging your weight loss process, or it could even be the main cause of your abdominal fat gain.

Overeating and Bingeing: When you don't have a regular eating schedule, it's easy to become overly hungry, leading to overeating or bingeing when you finally do eat. This often results in consuming more calories than your body needs.

Disrupted Metabolism: A consistent eating schedule helps keep your metabolism stable. Irregular eating patterns can disrupt your metabolism, leading to inefficiencies in how your body processes and uses energy, potentially resulting in increased fat storage.

Blood Sugar Fluctuations: Eating at inconsistent times can cause spikes and crashes in blood sugar levels, which can lead to increased hunger and cravings for sugary or high-carb foods.

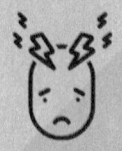

Increased Stress and Cortisol Levels: Irregular eating can cause stress due to fluctuating energy levels and uncertainty about when or what to eat next. Elevated stress can increase cortisol levels, a hormone linked to fat accumulation, particularly around the abdomen.

Disrupted Sleep: Irregular eating patterns can affect sleep, especially if you're eating late at night. Poor sleep is associated with hormonal imbalances that can increase hunger and cravings, contributing to weight gain.

How to fix this?

The first step is to accept that your metabolism needs a pattern to optimize internal biochemical reactions. Make a commitment to establish fixed times for your meals.

Have the discipline to distribute your meal portions throughout the day in a way that is convenient and comfortable for you and adapted to your routine.

- If necessary, divide or group meals at specific times of the day.

- Try to maintain consistency in the quality and calorie content of these meals. Ideally, you should consume exactly the same foods to avoid unexpected insulin spikes.

- Create a well-defined eating routine and stay focused, as constantly creating insulin spikes through disordered meals at different times will cause your metabolism to tend to directly store this extra energy in the form of fat.

tip n° 21
Creatine benefits and how to use it

Let's talk about the most studied and well-known food supplement in the world. With proven effects at all levels of modern research and highly recommended for men and women of all ages. Creatine is extremely well-known in the world of sports for its rapid results in terms of physical strength and muscular endurance, but its benefits extend far beyond bodybuilding.

- **Increased Muscle Mass:** Creatine can help increase muscle size by drawing water into muscle cells and supporting protein synthesis.

- **Improved Strength and Power:** It boosts the energy available to muscles during intense exercise, allowing you to lift heavier and perform better in high-intensity workouts.

- **Enhanced Workout Performance:** Creatine can extend your workout duration and intensity, enabling you to do more sets.

- **Faster Recovery:** It can reduce muscle damage and soreness, helping you recover quicker and get back to training sooner.

- **Supports Fat Loss:** By allowing you to work out harder and longer, creatine can indirectly help with fat loss through increased calorie burn and metabolism.

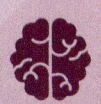

- **Potential Cognitive Benefits:** Some studies suggest that creatine may improve brain function and reduce mental fatigue during demanding tasks.

When you take creatine, it increases the amount of stored energy in your muscles, allowing you to lift heavier weights or work out for longer periods. This extra energy can lead to bigger gains in muscle mass, which is great because having more muscle means you burn more calories even when you're not working out. It's like turning your body into a calorie-burning machine!

Creatine can also help with weight loss by enhancing your workout performance. If you're able to exercise with more intensity or for longer, you'll burn more calories, which can aid in losing fat. Additionally, creatine can improve recovery time, allowing you to stick to your fitness routine without feeling too sore or exhausted.

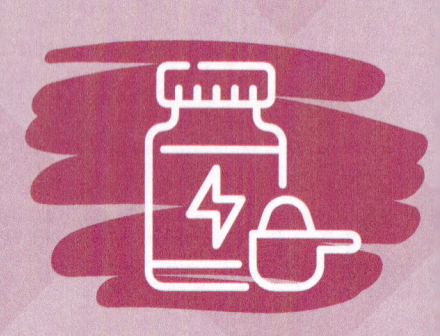

Creatine is a natural compound that your body produces and is also found in some foods. It helps provide energy to your muscles during high-intensity exercise. You can get more creatine in your diet by eating creatine-rich foods like:

- **Red Meat:** Beef and lamb are rich in creatine.
- **Fish:** Salmon, tuna, and herring are good sources.
- **Pork:** Pork chops and tenderloins contain creatine.

To supplement with creatine: start by taking 3-5 grams once a day. If you're new to creatine, some people choose to do a "loading phase," where they take 20 grams daily (split into 4 doses) for 5-7 days to saturate muscles quickly. Afterward, or if you skip the loading phase, maintain 3-5 grams daily, ideally after a workout.

tip n° 22 Mini-bulking strategy

Imagine you've been following a weight loss plan for a few weeks, eating healthier, and working out regularly. At first, you see great results: the numbers on the scale are going down, your clothes are fitting better, and you're feeling more energized. But then, all of a sudden, the progress stops. You step on the scale, and it hasn't budged for a few days or even weeks. You start to wonder what's happening because you're still eating right and exercising.
Yes, you have reached a plateau again!

In this situation, your body might have adapted to your current routine, so it's not burning as many calories as before. It can be frustrating because you're doing everything "right," but it feels like you're stuck in place. Hitting a plateau is common in weight loss journeys, and it's your body's way of saying it's time for a change. To break through it, you might need to switch up your workout routine, adjust your diet, or even get more sleep to give your body a little surprise and kickstart your progress again. Don't worry; it's part of the process, and with this advanced strategy, you'll be back on track in no time!

The **Mini-bulking strategy** consists of confusing your metabolism for a short period of time by consuming a high amount of calories again for a brief period of time (a few days) and then suddenly returning to the weight loss diet.

During this mini-bulking phase, you focus on strength training to encourage muscle growth while being careful not to overdo it with extra calories. Think of it as taking a short break from strict dieting to give your body the nutrients and energy it needs to grow muscle and get stronger.

Here's an example: for four weeks, you might add an extra 300-500 calories a day to your diet, coming from protein-rich foods like chicken, fish, or beans, and healthy carbs like whole grains and vegetables. You'll also increase your strength training sessions to build muscle. By the end of the mini-bulking phase, you might notice you're a bit heavier, but most of that extra weight is muscle, not fat. After this phase, you switch back to a lower-calorie diet to lose the extra fat you might have gained during mini-bulking. This way, you end up with more muscle, which helps burn more calories even when you're not working out, and you can continue with your weight loss process with more energy and strength. Overall, the mini-bulking strategy helps balance muscle growth and fat loss, keeping your metabolism active and your body strong.

And, as your metabolism ends up adapting to the new phase of high calorie consumption for a brief period of time, when you return to the calorie restriction phase, your body loses fat again much more efficiently than before.

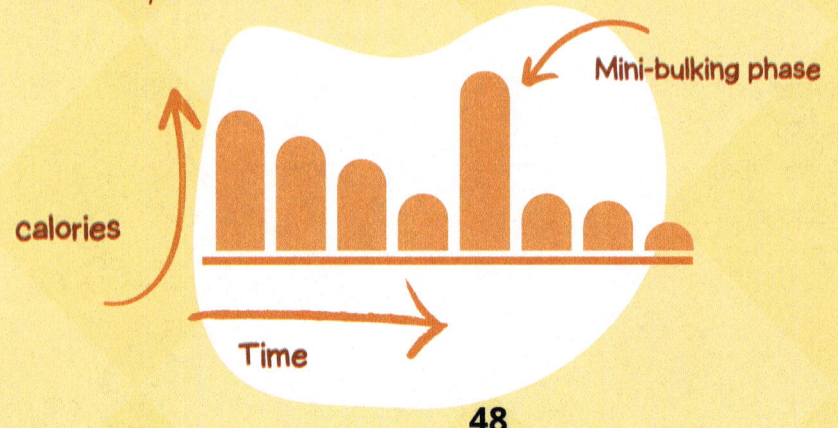

tip n° 23 Calcium supplementation

Let's talk now about one of the best-known minerals and cheapest dietary supplements, but which can greatly impact your results with fat loss and muscle mass gain. A calcium-poor diet can make it harder for us to lose weight for a few reasons. Let's break it down

Reduced Fat Metabolism: Calcium plays a role in regulating fat metabolism. When calcium intake is low, it can affect your body's ability to break down fat, leading to slower fat loss. Studies have shown that sufficient calcium intake can support the breakdown of fat cells, promoting weight loss.

Muscle Weakness: Calcium is involved in muscle contraction and relaxation. A lack of calcium can lead to muscle weakness or cramps, impacting your ability to exercise effectively. If your workouts are less intense or frequent due to muscle issues, it can slow down your weight loss progress

Imbalanced Hormones: Calcium deficiency can affect hormone levels, including those that regulate appetite and metabolism. This imbalance could lead to increased hunger, cravings, or slower metabolism, which may make it harder to lose weight.

In summary, it is important to highlight that the mineral calcium does not have thermogenic properties to enhance your fat loss alone, unlike other substances that we have already presented and will present here. However a diet low in calcium can make it harder to lose weight because it can affect your body's ability to burn fat and keep your bones and muscles strong. To stay on track with your weight loss goals, aim to include calcium-rich foods like dairy products (milk, cheese, yogurt), leafy greens, and fortified foods (like certain juices and cereals) in your meals.

Dosage and daily recommendation

Calcium supplementation can be a helpful way to ensure you're getting enough calcium, especially if your diet doesn't provide enough of this important mineral. If you're considering a calcium supplement, aim for a dosage that meets your daily requirements without exceeding the recommended limits. For most adults, the daily calcium intake should be about 1,000 mg to 1,200 mg. However, don't forget to count the calcium you're getting from food sources like dairy products, leafy greens, and fortified foods. If you're unsure about your calcium needs, it's a good idea to talk to a healthcare provider or nutritionist, as they can guide you on the right dosage and type of supplement to take. Remember, taking too much calcium can lead to other health issues, so moderation is key!

tip nº 24
HIIT - Advanced fat loss Strategy

If you are already engaged in a routine of physical activities focused on fat loss but are feeling that the results are still appearing slowly or are almost stagnating on a plateau again, pay attention because this tip will change the whole game for you.

HIIT is one of the most advanced cardio techniques known today. Widely used by high-level athletes, HIIT (stands for "High-Intensity Interval Training) is proven to be able to burn fat in a much more intense and faster way than other common exercise strategies.

Recently conducted studies have shown that after a HIIT session our metabolism remains in "fat burning" mode for up to <u>9 hours after</u> completing the series, which is simply incredible!

How to perform HIIT correctly?

First, let's understand the basic idea behind HIIT: you're going to do short bursts of high-intensity exercise, followed by brief periods of rest or low-intensity activity. The goal is to get your heart rate up and then give your body a chance to recover before the next burst. Here's a simple way to get started:

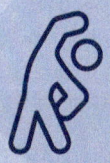

Warm-Up: Begin with a 5-minute warm-up to get your body ready for action. You can do light jogging, brisk walking, or some gentle stretches.

Pick Your Exercises: For beginners, let's start with basic moves like jumping jacks, high knees, bodyweight squats, or push-ups. Choose three or four exercises you feel comfortable with.

Set the Timer: For beginners, let's do 20 seconds of high-intensity exercise, followed by 40 seconds of rest or light activity. You can use a timer app on your phone to keep track.

Start the HIIT Circuit: Do your first exercise (like jumping jacks) for 20 seconds as fast as you can while maintaining good form. Then rest for 40 seconds, either by standing still or walking around to catch your breath.

Repeat and Rotate: After your rest, move on to the next exercise, and repeat the same pattern: 20 seconds of intensity, 40 seconds of rest. Continue this for 10-15 minutes, depending on your comfort level.

Cool Down: Once you've completed your HIIT circuit, take 5 minutes to cool down. Walk around, do some light stretching, and focus on slowing your breathing.

tip n° 25

The benefits of Omega 3

Omega-3 is a fatty acid with a great impact on muscle synthesis and fat metabolism. An omega-3 deficiency can lead to increased inflammation, reduced muscle growth, and hindered fat metabolism, making it harder to lose weight and gain muscle effectively.

Do you have a diet low in omega 3?

- **Fatty Fish:** Salmon, mackerel, sardines, herring, trout, and anchovies are among the richest sources of omega-3.

- **Chia Seeds:** These tiny seeds are high in omega-3, specifically ALA (alpha-linolenic acid).

- **Flaxseeds:** Another plant-based source of omega-3, flaxseeds are commonly ground into flaxseed meal or used as flaxseed oil.

- **Walnuts:** These nuts contain a good amount of omega-3, making them a healthy snack or addition to meals.

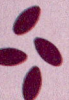

- **Hemp Seeds:** These seeds contain both omega-3 and omega-6 fatty acids in beneficial ratios.

- **Soybeans:** Soy-based products like tofu and edamame contain moderate amounts of omega-3.

Benefits directly associated with Omega 3

Supports Fat Loss: Omega-3 has been shown to help reduce body fat. It can boost your metabolism, making it easier for your body to burn calories efficiently. Additionally, omega-3 can reduce the storage of fat in adipose tissue, leading to a decrease in overall body fat.

Improves Insulin Sensitivity: Omega-3 can enhance insulin sensitivity, which helps regulate blood sugar levels. This can prevent spikes in blood sugar that might lead to increased fat storage, making it easier to maintain a healthy weight.

Enhances Muscle Protein Synthesis: Omega-3 can support muscle protein synthesis, the process by which muscles grow and repair. This is crucial for muscle gain, especially when combined with resistance training and adequate protein intake.

Supports Heart Health: Omega-3 contributes to heart health by reducing bad cholesterol (LDL), increasing good cholesterol (HDL), and lowering blood pressure. A healthy heart can lead to better workout performance and overall health, supporting long-term fitness goals.

Dosage and how to supplement with Omega 3

The recommended daily dosage of omega-3 varies, but most health experts suggest a total of <u>250-500 milligrams </u>of combined EPA (eicosapentaenoic acid) and DHA (docosahexaenoic acid).

tip n° 26
Reducing waist volume with stomach vacuum

In addition to eliminating visceral and abdominal fat, and water retention and swelling (which we will discuss later), there is a very interesting and simple exercise to reduce the volume of the waist, leaving the body more harmonious and further highlighting the reduction in abdominal volume.

Stomach vacuum is an simple exercise to strengthen the internal muscles of the abdomen, especially the transversus abdominis and is widely used by bodybuilders and models to achieve a very slim waist appearance.

1. **Start Position**: You can perform this exercise standing, sitting, or lying on your back. Make sure your back is straight and you're comfortable.

2. **Exhale Deeply**: Begin by exhaling as much air as possible from your lungs. Really focus on pushing all the air out.

3. **Suck In Your Stomach**: After you've exhaled, suck your stomach in as far as possible. Imagine trying to touch your belly button to your spine. This creates a hollowing effect in your stomach.

4. **Hold the Position**: Hold this "sucked in" position for about 15 to 20 seconds to start. As you get more practiced, you can hold for longer, up to 60 seconds or more.

5. **Release and Breathe**: Relax your muscles and breathe normally for a few seconds as a break before repeating the exercise.

6. **Repeat**: Do about 3-5 repetitions of this exercise. As it gets easier, you can increase the number of repetitions.

The vacuum exercise is crucial because it strengthens the often-neglected inner abdominal muscles. Over time, if these muscles aren't strengthened, they can weaken and fail to properly support the viscera and internal organs. This lack of support can significantly increase belly volume. Additionally, fat accumulation can exacerbate this issue, making it even more important to maintain these core muscles.

Performing the stomach vacuum daily can help improve core strength and reduce your waist size over time, giving your abdomen a flatter appearance. It's a subtle exercise, so it's easy to do almost anywhere and anytime.

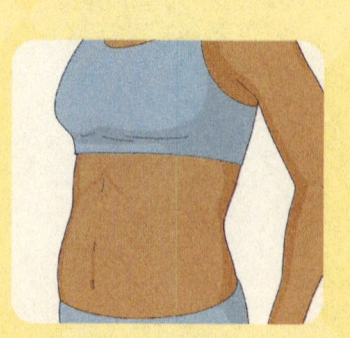

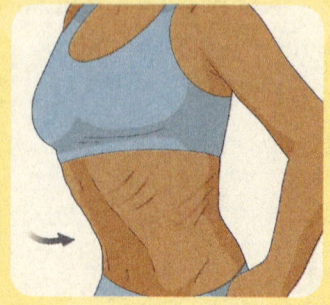

tip n° 27
Fix your sleep routine

When you don't get enough sleep or have disrupted sleep, it throws off your body's balance in a few important ways. One of the main things that happens is that your hormones go out of whack. There's a hormone called leptin, which helps you feel full, and another called ghrelin, which makes you feel hungry. When you don't sleep well, your body produces less leptin and more ghrelin, leading to increased hunger and cravings, especially for high-calorie and sugary foods.

In addition to this, when you're not sleeping enough, your body may not process sugar and carbohydrates as efficiently, which can lead to higher blood sugar levels and more fat storage. This can contribute to weight gain over time.

Increased Fat Storage: Poor sleep can raise cortisol levels, which can lead to more fat storage, particularly around the belly area.

Mood Swings and Stress: Poor sleep can make you irritable and stressed, leading to emotional eating and other habits that hinder weight loss. Studies have shown a strong link between stress levels and weight gain.

Reduced Muscle Recovery: Sleep is when your body repairs muscles. Without enough sleep, your muscles don't recover as quickly, which can limit muscle growth.

Slower Metabolism: When you don't get enough sleep, your body's metabolism can slow down, which means you burn fewer calories throughout the day.

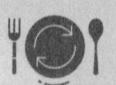

Increased Hunger: Poor sleep messes with the hormones that control hunger, making you crave more food, especially unhealthy snacks and sweets. This can make it harder to stick to a weight loss plan.

A study published in "Biological Psychiatry" found that stress-induced cortisol secretion was associated with higher calorie intake and weight gain. Similarly, research in the "American Journal of Epidemiology" showed that chronic stress could increase the risk of developing obesity.

.To fix this and optimize fat loss, try these simple tips for better sleep:

1. **Establish a Sleep Routine**: Go to bed and wake up at the same time every day to regulate your body's internal clock.
2. **Avoid Caffeine and Heavy Meals Late**: Try not to consume caffeine or eat heavy meals in the evening, as they can disrupt sleep. Caffeine stays active in your body for a few hours after you drink it, but the exact time can vary. On average, it takes about 3 to 5 hours for half of the caffeine to be processed and start to leave your system. However, it can range from 1.5 to 9.5 hours, depending on things like age, genetics, and overall health.
3. **Exercise Regularly**: Regular physical activity can help you sleep better, but try to avoid intense workouts right before bed as this can trigger a state of alert, raising body temperature, heart rate and high levels of adrenaline.

tip n° 28
The impact of leg training

At this stage, you already understand the importance of performing physical exercises to optimize your progress, whether your priorities are gaining muscle or losing fat, or even both.

However, if we were to consider a type of workout as one of the best and most efficient for boosting your progress, it would certainly be everything that includes leg exercises.

But why specifically the legs? Physical exercises, mainly with weights, performed with the legs are one of the best known ways to stimulate the production of endogenous testosterone, while we also spend a lot of calories with these exercises.

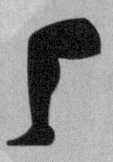

Large Muscle Groups: Your legs contain some of the largest muscle groups in the body, such as the quadriceps, hamstrings, glutes, and calves. When you work these muscles, you burn more calories during exercise because bigger muscles require more energy.

Increased Metabolism: Because leg exercises engage large muscle groups, they can boost your metabolism. This means you'll continue to burn more calories even after your workout, a phenomenon known as the "afterburn effect" or excess post-exercise oxygen consumption (EPOC).

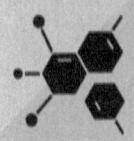

Hormonal Response: Intense leg workouts can stimulate the release of growth hormones and testosterone, which are essential for muscle growth. The increased production of these hormones helps with muscle building and can contribute to fat loss by improving muscle-to-fat ratio.

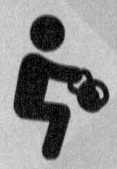

Functional Movement: Leg exercises often involve compound movements (exercises that work multiple muscle groups at once), such as squats, lunges, and deadlifts. These exercises not only build muscle but also improve functional strength, balance, and coordination, which are important for overall fitness and daily activities.

High Caloric Burn: Because leg workouts are typically more intense and involve larger muscle groups, they burn more calories compared to exercises targeting smaller muscles. This helps with weight loss by increasing overall energy expenditure.

We know that leg training can be the most physically demanding, requiring good respiratory capacity and the development of several accessory muscle groups.

In summary, leg exercise is one of your best options for weight loss and muscle gain because they target large muscle groups, boost metabolism, promote the release of muscle-building hormones, and burn way more calories. Not neglecting the importance of stimulating your leg muscles will certainly accelerate your results in weight loss and lean mass gain.

tip n° 29
Accelerate your results with caffeine

Caffeine isn't just your morning pick-me-up; it's a secret weapon in your fat-loss arsenal! Whether you're sipping on coffee or enjoying a cup of tea, caffeine can supercharge your metabolism and speed up the rate at which your body burns calories, even without exercising. In this chapter, we're diving into all the ways caffeine can help you burn more fat, keep your appetite in check, and stay energized on your weight loss journey. Get ready to discover how this powerful stimulant can rev up your results and make those stubborn pounds disappear!

Caffeine is an interesting component with thermogenic properties that can boost weight loss by increasing metabolism, enhancing fat oxidation, suppressing appetite, and providing extra energy for more intense workouts.

Caffeine has been found to increase the body's ability to break down stored fat and use it as a source of energy, a process known as fat oxidation. When you consume caffeine, it stimulates the release of adrenaline, a hormone that signals your body to release fatty acids into the bloodstream. These fatty acids can then be used as fuel by your muscles, especially during exercise.
This process is particularly beneficial for weight loss because it encourages your body to utilize fat stores for energy rather than relying solely on carbohydrates. This not only helps in reducing body fat but also provides an energy boost for workouts, allowing you to exercise longer and with greater intensity.

Studies have shown that caffeine can significantly increase the rate of <u>fat oxidation during both rest and exercise</u>, making it a valuable tool for those aiming to lose weight. This enhanced fat-burning capability, combined with its other benefits like boosting metabolism and increasing exercise performance, makes caffeine a popular ingredient in many weight loss and pre-workout supplements. However, it's important to use caffeine in moderation to avoid side effects such as anxiety, increased heart rate, or disrupted sleep.

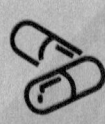

Know Your Limits: For most adults, a safe daily limit of caffeine is about <u>400 milligrams</u>. This is roughly the amount in four 8-ounce cups of brewed coffee or about 10 cans of cola. Keep in mind that sensitivity to caffeine varies, so it's best to start with a lower dose to see how it affects you.

Time Your Intake: To avoid sleep disruptions, try not to consume caffeine late in the day. A good rule of thumb is to stop drinking caffeinated beverages after 2 or 3 p.m.

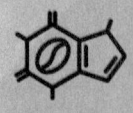

Start Slowly: If you're new to caffeine or haven't used it in a while, begin with a lower dose, such as 100 to 200 milligrams, and gradually increase if needed. This will help you gauge your body's response without overdoing it.

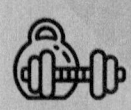

Use Before Workouts: For a performance boost, consider consuming caffeine about 30 to 60 minutes before exercise. This timing allows it to take effect, giving you more energy and focus during your workout.

Stay Hydrated: Caffeine can have a mild diuretic effect, so make sure to drink plenty of water throughout the day to stay hydrated.

tip n° 30
Advanced training strategy - Resting pause

If you feel that your weight training is no longer yielding the same results as before, you can try changing your training technique. A new stimulus will positively impact your progress after a few months of performing the same exercise repetition pattern.

Resting-pause is an advanced technique where you will divide a series into at least 3 phases and intersperse them with brief seconds of rest.

The result is that you will have a much greater caloric expenditure while taking your muscles beyond extreme failure. If you've never tried this strategy before, you can get quick results after just a few weeks.

- **Start with a Weighty Lift**: Choose a weight that's heavy enough to challenge you. Perform your set, for example, doing as many reps as you can until you can't do another rep properly.

- **Short Rest**: Instead of ending your set there, take a very short break — usually around 10 to 20 seconds.

- **Go Again**: After the break, lift the same weight again for as many reps as you can manage.

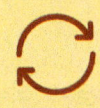

- **Repeat**: You can repeat this process a couple of times within the same set. This might mean doing a few more reps with short breaks in between each mini-set.

This technique works by allowing you to do more reps with a heavy weight than you would normally manage in one go, intensifying the training and stimulating more muscle growth and increasing total caloric expenditure. It's like squeezing out every last drop of strength and endurance from your muscles, making them work harder and potentially grow bigger!

Swapping your basic sets and reps for this simple advanced technique can provide huge advances in your conditioning and fitness.

Increased Muscle Activation: Allowing brief recovery periods within sets enables performing more reps with heavy weights, which intensifies muscle workload and promotes growth.

Boosted Metabolism: Intense lifting with short rests keeps your heart rate elevated, increasing your metabolic rate which continues to burn calories long after your workout, aiding fat loss.

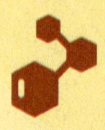

Greater Hormonal Response: The significant stress placed on your muscles can lead to increased production of muscle-building hormones like growth hormone and testosterone, essential for muscle repair and growth.

Improved Endurance: This technique helps enhance muscular endurance, as your muscles adapt to quick recovery and sustained effort.

tip n° 31 — Experience the benefits of green tea

Another highly studied natural extract with conclusive results on helping to lose fat is green tea.
Just like black tea, it is a powerful natural thermogenic, with caffeine and very rich in antioxidants, which certainly represents a potential ally in your fat loss process.

Both green tea and black tea come from the same plant, Camellia sinensis, but the main difference is in their processing: green tea is made from unoxidized leaves, keeping its delicate flavor and high catechin content, while black tea is fully oxidized, which gives it a darker color and a richer, more robust taste.

Green tea deserves a special position in this content because, due to the fact that it is less oxidized, it contains a high dose of catechins, such as epigallocatechin gallate (EGCG), that boost metabolism and promote fat oxidation, helping to burn more calories even when you are at rest.

Together, the phytoactive compounds present in green tea help in practically all aspects of weight loss, such as appetite suppression, thermogenesis, fat oxidation and fat metabolism.
Some studies suggest that catechins may reduce the absorption of dietary fat, potentially lowering overall fat intake. This effect, combined with increased metabolism, can lead to a gradual reduction in body fat.

Catechins (EGCG)

- **Metabolism Boost**: Catechins, particularly Epigallocatechin Gallate (EGCG), help boost metabolism by increasing the body's energy expenditure, which means you burn more calories even when at rest.

- **Fat Oxidation**: EGCG can promote fat oxidation, encouraging the body to break down fat cells and use them as energy.

- **Thermogenesis**: Catechins can increase thermogenesis, the process of generating heat in the body, which helps burn calories.

- **Energy Boost**: Caffeine in green tea extract provides a quick energy boost, helping you feel more alert and focused. This can be especially useful for getting through workouts.

- **Appetite Suppression**: Green tea extract can also help suppress appetite, potentially reducing calorie intake throughout the day.

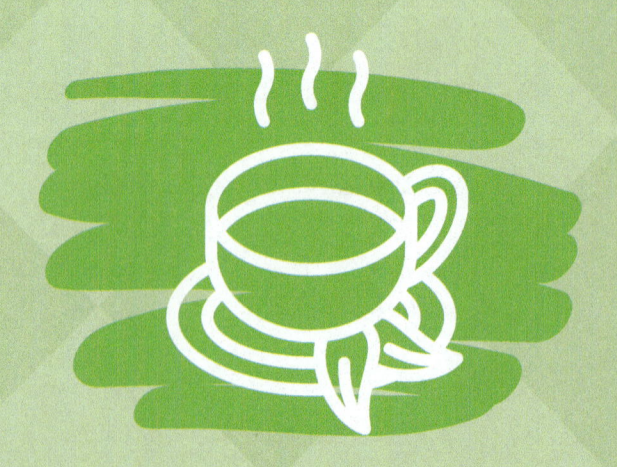

tip n° 32
Eliminating water retention

Some of the total weight you see on the scale when evaluating your results is actually water retention. This effect may be causing a bloated appearance, leaving your skin thicker and your muscles less visible, causing the impression that you have more fat than you actually do.

Water retention and bloating can be caused by various factors, including high sodium intake, hormonal changes, dehydration, certain medications, or underlying health conditions, which lead to the body retaining excess fluids, often resulting in swelling and discomfort.

Fortunately, there are simple and effective ways to get around this situation. You can apply some of these adjustments in the short term to promote a more "Slim" appearance for a short period of time, or permanently adjust your diet to reduce the effects of water retention as much as possible.

- **Reduce Sodium Intake:** Too much salt can cause your body to retain water. Cut down on salty foods like processed snacks and fast food.

- **Stay Hydrated:** It might sound counterintuitive, but drinking more water can help flush out excess fluids. Aim for at least 8 cups of water a day.

Eat Potassium-Rich Foods: Foods like bananas, avocados, and sweet potatoes contain potassium, which can help balance sodium levels and reduce water retention.

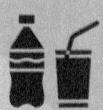

Limit Carbonated Drinks: Fizzy drinks can lead to gas and bloating, so opt for still water or herbal teas instead.

Consider Herbal Teas: Teas like dandelion, ginger, or peppermint are known for their diuretic properties, which can help reduce bloating.

Bodybuilders and models sometimes use a dehydration process to temporarily eliminate water retention, creating a more defined and toned appearance for competitions or photo shoots. Here's an easy explanation of how it works:

To create that "ripped" or "cut" look, they follow specific techniques to shed excess water from their bodies.

1. **Reduce Sodium Intake**: Sodium (salt) makes your body retain water. By cutting down on sodium-rich foods, bodybuilders and models aim to minimize water retention.
2. **Carb Depletion and Loading**: Carbohydrates can lead to water retention because they are stored with water in the muscles. Then, before the event, they might reduce carb intake.
3. **Increased Water Intake, Then Restriction**: In the days leading up to an event, they might drink extra water to signal the body to flush out excess fluids. A day or two before the event, they cut back on water intake to create a temporary dehydration effect.

tip nº 33 Forskolin Extract

Forskolin extract comes from the roots of the Coleus forskohlii plant, which is native to South Asia. It's used in traditional Ayurvedic medicine and has gained popularity as a supplement, mainly for its benefits in weight loss and in muscle development.

As a supplement, Forskolin extract is available in various formats, including capsules, tablets, powder, and liquid extracts, providing multiple options for users to choose from based on their preference, with capsules and tablets being the most common.

Forskolin extract is also believed to promote muscle growth, making it popular among bodybuilders. Some studies suggest that it can help increase lean body mass while reducing body fat.

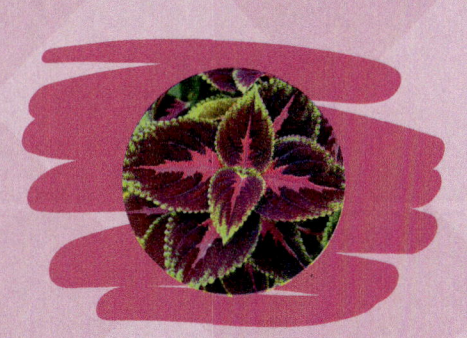

Despite being a relatively recent supplement on the market and still having several studies underway to determine all the benefits, Forskolin has already attracted the attention of athletes and people looking to improve their physical condition.

Boosts Fat Breakdown: Forskolin increases levels of a molecule called cyclic AMP (cAMP), which can activate enzymes that break down stored fat, making it easier for the body to burn fat for energy.

Promotes Muscle Gain: By stimulating cAMP, forskolin might also encourage muscle growth, helping you build lean muscle mass while losing fat.

Supports Metabolism: Higher cAMP levels can boost metabolism, potentially leading to increased calorie burning and more efficient weight loss.

Improves Blood Sugar Regulation: cAMP is involved in insulin secretion and glucose metabolism, helping to maintain stable blood sugar levels, which is key for overall health and energy.

- **Dosage**: A common dosage for forskolin supplements is 250 mg of an extract standardized to 10-20% forskolin, taken 1-2 times a day. This standardized percentage ensures you're getting a consistent amount of the active compound.

- **Timing**: Forskolin supplements are usually taken on an empty stomach, either 15-30 minutes before a meal or in the morning before breakfast.

- **With Water**: Always take forskolin with a full glass of water to aid in absorption and reduce the risk of stomach upset.

tip n° 34
Recipe idea
Protein dessert

Banana Berry Whey Protein Smoothie

This smoothie is packed with protein from the whey protein powder, vitamins, and antioxidants from the fruits. It's a satisfying way to refuel after a workout or to start your day on a healthy note.

Ingredients:

- 1 ripe banana
- 1/2 cup mixed berries (such as strawberries, blueberries, raspberries)
- 1 scoop of vanilla whey protein powder
- 1 cup unsweetened almond milk (or any milk of your choice)
- 1 tablespoon honey or maple syrup (optional, for added sweetness)
- Ice cubes (optional, for a colder smoothie)

Instructions:

Peel the banana and break it into smaller chunks.

Wash the mixed berries thoroughly.

In a blender, combine the banana chunks, mixed berries, vanilla whey protein powder, almond milk, and honey or maple syrup (if using).

If desired, add a few ice cubes to make the smoothie colder.

Blend all the ingredients together until smooth and creamy. Taste the smoothie and adjust the sweetness level by adding more honey or maple syrup if needed.

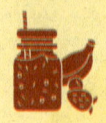

Enjoy your Banana Berry Whey Protein Smoothie immediately as a post-workout snack or a quick breakfast!

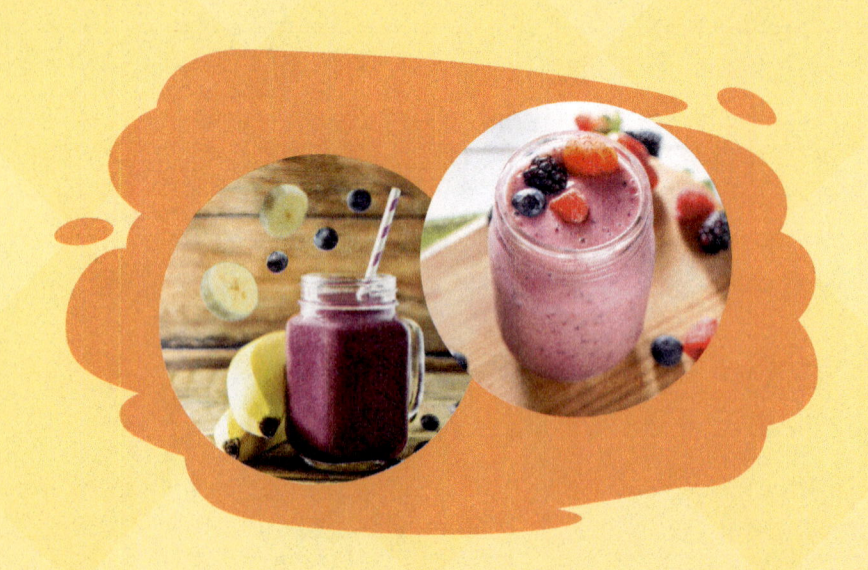

tip n° 35
Try Chitosan for appetite reduction

If you suspect that your regular diet may be loaded with bad fats, or that cholesterol is sabotaging both your health and fitness, perhaps this chapter will provide a powerful weapon for you to fight against excess fat.

<u>Chitosan</u> is a natural substance derived from the shells of crustaceans like shrimp, crab, and lobster. It's a type of fiber that has the unique ability to bind with fat and cholesterol in the digestive system, making it a recent but increasingly popular supplement for those interested in weight loss and better heart health.

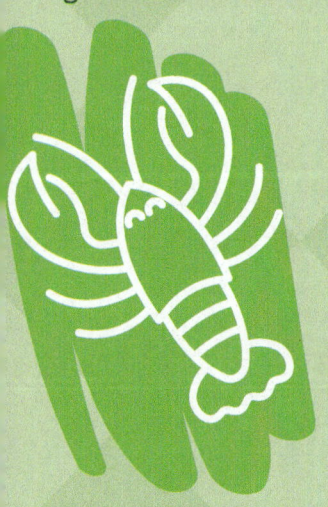

<u>Here's how chitosan works</u>: once ingested, it moves through the digestive system and binds to dietary fats, preventing them from being absorbed into the bloodstream. Instead, these bound fats are carried out of the body, which can help reduce calorie intake and support weight loss. This fat-binding ability has made chitosan a favorite among people looking for a natural approach to managing their weight.

Chitosan has other benefits too. By limiting the absorption of fat, it can also help lower cholesterol levels, which is great for heart health. Since it's a type of fiber, chitosan can also aid digestion and promote better gut health.

Besides its effects on fat and cholesterol, some studies suggest chitosan might help with wound healing and support the immune system, offering additional health benefits.

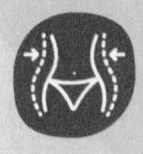

Weight Loss Help: Chitosan can bind to dietary fats in your digestive system, preventing them from being absorbed. This means those fats don't get stored in your body, which can help you lose weight or manage your current weight.

Lower Cholesterol: Because chitosan can capture fats, it can also help reduce cholesterol levels. This is good news for your heart, as lower cholesterol means a reduced risk of heart disease.

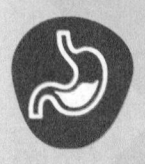

Improved Digestion: As a type of fiber, chitosan can support a healthy digestive system. It can help keep things moving smoothly and might even contribute to a healthier gut.

- **When to Take It**: The best time to take chitosan is before meals. This way, it can bind to the fats in the food you're about to eat, helping to reduce the amount of fat absorbed by your body.
- **Dosage**: A common dose is 1 to 2 grams of chitosan per day, divided into smaller doses. For example, you might take 500 mg before each meal, which adds up to 1.5 grams daily. Some people might need more or less, so it's a good idea to start on the lower end and adjust as needed.
- **With Water**: Chitosan is a type of fiber, so it's important to take it with plenty of water to help it move through your digestive system and do its job. Drink a full glass of water with each dose.

tip nº 36
Ketogenic diet and fat consumption

One of the most prominent diet modalities that has become famous and aroused a lot of interest is the ketogenic diet. But after all, what does science confirm about the ketogenic diet?

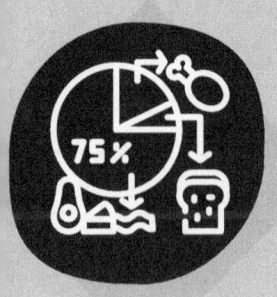

A ketogenic diet, often just called "keto," is a way of eating that focuses on very low carbs, moderate protein, and high good quality fat. The goal is to get your body into a state called "ketosis," where it starts using fat for energy instead of carbohydrates.

Normally, your body gets energy from carbs like bread, pasta, and sugar. But when you cut way back on carbs, your body eventually starts breaking down fat into substances called "ketones," which it uses for energy. This shift can help with weight loss and may have other health benefits, like stabilizing blood sugar and reducing cravings.

In a typical ketogenic diet you'd avoid high-carb foods like bread, rice, potatoes, and sweets and consume larger portions of foods such as:

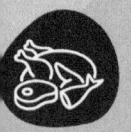

Protein Sources
- **Meat**: Beef, pork, lamb, chicken, turkey
- **Fish**: Salmon, mackerel, sardines, tuna
- **Eggs**: Whole eggs from any source

Fats and Oils

- Avocado and avocado oil
- Olive oil
- Coconut oil
- Butter
- Ghee

Dairy

- Cheese: Cheddar, mozzarella, Parmesan, cream cheese
- Heavy cream
- Full-fat Greek yogurt (in moderation)

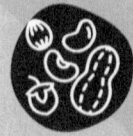

Nuts and Seeds

- Almonds, walnuts, pecans, hazelnuts
- Chia seeds, flaxseeds, sunflower seeds, pumpkin seeds

The ketogenic diet was born out of contradiction, as people used to think that to lose fat, we should stay away from foods rich in fat.

However, we know that <u>foods rich in good fats</u> can very well be implemented in a calorie-restricted diet focused on weight loss.

The real villains of weight loss are low quality fats and carbohydrates, especially those with higher glycemic indexes. This is because they are easily digested and assimilated by the body, unlike proteins and good fats, which require a lot of work to be metabolized.

tip n° 37
Boost your results with Ephedrine

Another compound that you can use to boost your fat burning results is Ephedrine. It has a proven and studied impact on weight loss and the treatment of obesity, and is even used as medication for this purpose. However, ephedrine-based products are regulated in many countries, including the U.S. and Canada. Always check the legality and safety of these products in your country, and consult a healthcare professional before using them.

Ephedrine is a chemical compound derived from the Ephedra plant, traditionally used in Chinese medicine. Known for its stimulating effects, which can be similar to adrenaline. It's been used in various weight loss products because it can boost energy, suppress appetite, and potentially increase metabolism, making it easier to burn calories and reduce body fat.

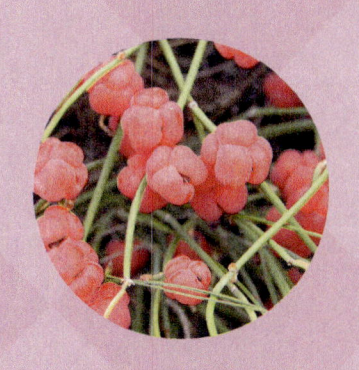

Just like the other natural extracts and supplements that we explain throughout this material, use Ephedrine as a complement to your efforts in your diet and training routine. We are talking about a compound with even stronger thermogenic properties than most of the others we have explained so far, so think of ephedrine as a last resort and check availability in your country.

Appetite Suppressant: One of the primary reasons ephedrine is used in weight loss products is its ability to reduce hunger. By suppressing appetite, it helps you feel fuller for longer, making it easier to stick to a calorie-controlled diet. This can be particularly useful for people who struggle with frequent snacking or emotional eating.

Metabolism Booster: Ephedrine stimulates the body's metabolism, increasing the rate at which calories are burned. This thermogenic effect can lead to greater fat loss over time, as your body uses more energy even at rest. It can also increase heat production, which is why it's often included in fat-burning supplements.

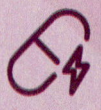

Energy Enhancer: Because of its stimulating properties, ephedrine can provide an energy boost, which can be beneficial for workouts and daily activities. This added energy can motivate you to exercise more intensely or for longer periods, contributing to increased calorie expenditure and muscle tone.

How to take and safe dosage

A typical dose for adults is 25 to 50 milligrams of ephedrine, taken every 4 to 6 hours. It's crucial not to exceed 150 milligrams in a 24-hour period.

tip n° 38
Advanced training strategy - Pyramid

Returning to weight training, which is our greatest ally for gaining muscle volume and burn fat, let's now talk about a very challenging strategy, which will certainly make you progress or break a phase of stagnation in gaining muscle mass.

Unlike the Drop set strategy, which we discussed previously, in which we reduce the weights and perform several sets in a row, in the pyramid strategy, we will perform the exact opposite.

<u>Pyramid training</u> is an effective way to build muscle mass. The strategy gets its name from the shape of a pyramid because it starts with <u>light weights and high repetitions</u> at the base, then gradually moves to heavier weights and fewer repetitions at the top.

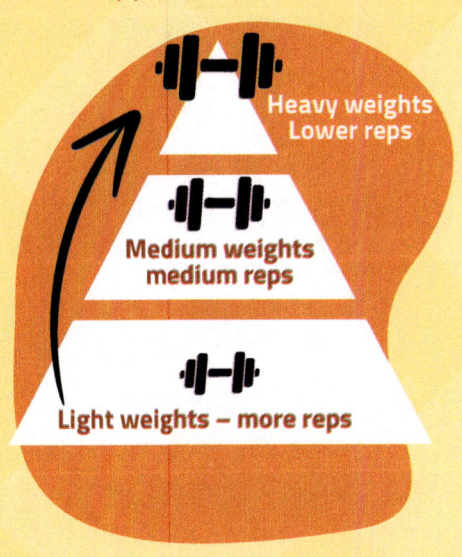

**Heavy weights
Lower reps**

**Medium weights
medium reps**

Light weights – more reps

This advanced training strategy will allow you to develop more strength and the ability to lift increasingly heavier **weights** over time, but it will also develop localized muscular endurance.

- **Begin Light**: Start with a lighter weight that you can lift comfortably for about 12 to 15 repetitions. This serves as a warm-up and helps you get into the rhythm of the exercise.

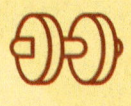

- **Increase Weight, Decrease Reps**: As you progress, increase the weight for the next set but reduce the number of repetitions. For example, you might go from 12 reps to 10 reps with a slightly heavier weight.

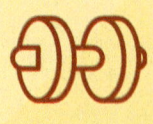

- **Go Heavier, Do Fewer Reps**: Keep adding more weight and lowering the repetitions with each set. The final set at the top of the pyramid is usually the heaviest, with just 4 to 6 repetitions. This is where you're pushing your muscles to their limits and stimulating muscle growth.

- **Rest and Repeat**: Once you reach the peak of the pyramid, you can repeat the process or work your way back down by decreasing the weight and increasing the repetitions, forming a complete pyramid shape.

Pyramid training is a great way to challenge your muscles, as it combines endurance and strength training in a single session.

What does science say about intervals between sets?

Studies suggest that for muscle hypertrophy (increase in muscle mass), rest intervals of 1 to 2 minutes between sets are ideal. This timing provides enough recovery while still stressing the muscles to promote growth, making it a good fit for bodybuilding and muscle-building workouts.

tip n° 39

Recipe idea
High protein lunch

Low Carb Protein Bowl

This recipe is versatile, satisfying, and packed with protein and healthy fats, making it an excellent option for a low-carb lunch. Feel free to customize it with your favorite low-carb veggies!

Ingredients:

- Grilled chicken breast, diced
- Avocado, sliced
- Mixed salad greens (spinach, kale, arugula, etc.)
- Cherry tomatoes, halved
- Cucumber, sliced
- Red onion, thinly sliced
- Feta cheese, crumbled
- Olive oil
- Lemon juice
- Salt and pepper to taste
- Optional: nuts (almonds, walnuts) for extra crunch

Instructions:

Start by grilling or baking the chicken breast until fully cooked. Season with salt, pepper, and your favorite spices.

While the chicken is cooking, prepare the salad ingredients. Wash and chop the salad greens, slice the avocado, cherry tomatoes, cucumber, and red onion.

In a small bowl, whisk together some olive oil, lemon juice, salt, and pepper to make a simple vinaigrette.

Once the chicken is done, let it cool slightly, then dice it into bite-sized pieces.

Assemble your protein bowl by layering the salad greens as the base, then adding the diced chicken, avocado slices, cherry tomatoes, cucumber, red onion, and crumbled feta cheese on top.
Drizzle the vinaigrette over the bowl.
Enjoy your delicious and nutritious low carb protein bowl!

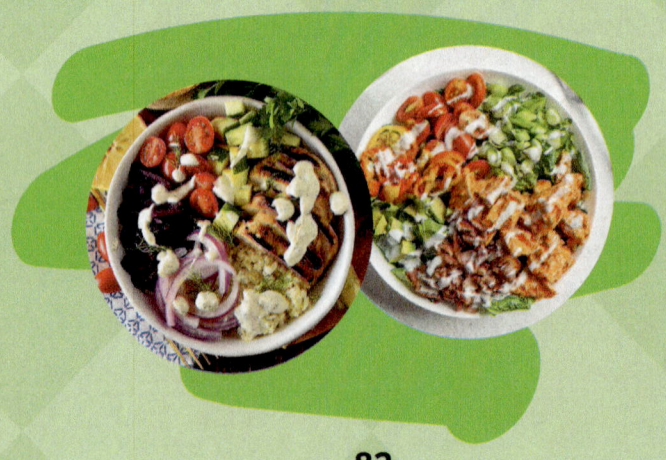

tip n° 40
Add safflower oil to your routine

Safflower oil might not be the first thing you think of when it comes to weight loss, but it's an interesting addition to your diet. This oil is derived from the seeds of the safflower plant, which is known for its vibrant orange and yellow flowers. What makes safflower oil unique is its high content of unsaturated fatty acids, particularly linoleic acid, which is an omega-6 fatty acid.

Helps with weight loss : safflower oil has gained attention because some studies strongly suggest it can help reduce body fat, especially around the midsection. It works by potentially promoting the breakdown of fat and enhancing muscle growth, making it a popular choice among those looking to lose weight and maintain muscle.

While safflower oil has some promising benefits, it's not a magic solution for weight loss. The key is to use it as part of a balanced diet and healthy lifestyle, focusing on portion control and regular exercise.

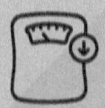

Aids in Fat Loss: Safflower oil contains linoleic acid, an omega-6 fatty acid that may help break down body fat, particularly around the belly area. This can be beneficial for individuals striving to shed excess weight and trim their waistlines.

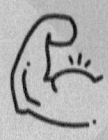

Supports Muscle Growth: Alongside its fat-burning properties, safflower oil has been linked to enhancing muscle growth since it's rich in linoleic acid, helping with muscle gain by promoting muscle protein synthesis and reducing inflammation.

Heart Health: Safflower oil is rich in unsaturated fats, which can help lower "bad" LDL cholesterol levels while increasing "good" HDL cholesterol. This heart-healthy profile may reduce the risk of cardiovascular diseases, providing an additional boost to overall well-being.

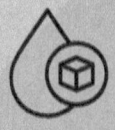

Balanced Blood Sugar: Some studies have shown that safflower oil consumption may aid in stabilizing blood sugar levels, which is crucial for managing weight and preventing insulin resistance.

Incorporating safflower oil into your diet for weight loss is simple and straightforward:

- **Quantity**: Aim to use about 1-2 tablespoons of safflower oil daily. This amount is enough to gain the health benefits without adding too many extra calories.

tip n° 41 — Optimize your fat loss with L-Carnitine

If you still want to test another commercially famous supplement specifically to help you enhance and accelerate fat loss, perhaps L-carnitine will be an interesting option for you.

L-carnitine is a naturally occurring amino acid derivative that plays a crucial role in the metabolism of fat. It works by transporting fatty acids into your cells' mitochondria, the "engines" within your cells that burn fats to create usable energy. This process is vital for burning fat and producing energy during workouts.

When it comes to weight loss, the main proven benefits of L-carnitine are its ability to help increase the body's efficiency in burning fat. This not only helps in reducing body weight but also improves endurance by keeping the body's energy stores efficiently replenished. Studies have shown that when combined with exercise, L-carnitine can lead to increased weight loss and improved muscle definition.

Additionally, L-carnitine can enhance the effectiveness of other weight loss practices like dieting by reducing the feeling of hunger and fatigue often associated with caloric restriction. Keep in mind that L-carnitine's benefits are most effective when it's used in conjunction with a healthy diet and regular exercise.

- **Enhances Fat Burning**: L-carnitine helps transport fats into the mitochondria of cells, where they are burned for energy, boosting your body's ability to burn fat and aiding in weight loss.
- **Increases Energy Levels**: By improving the efficiency of fat metabolism, L-carnitine can also increase energy levels, which can enhance performance and endurance during exercise.
- **Supports Heart Health**: Studies suggest that L-carnitine can support cardiovascular health by reducing blood pressure and the inflammatory process associated with heart disease.
- **Aids Muscle Recovery**: L-carnitine can reduce muscle soreness and damage after exercise, helping the body to recover faster.
- **Improves Brain Function**: Some research indicates that L-carnitine could have neuroprotective effects that help enhance brain function and cognition.

- **When to Take It**: L-carnitine is most effective when taken about 30 to 60 minutes before exercise. This timing helps maximize its fat-burning potential and can give you a bit more energy for your workout.
- **Daily Dosage**: A common dose of L-carnitine is between 500 mg to 2,000 mg per day. It's often recommended to start at the lower end of the scale to see how your body reacts and then adjust the dosage if needed.
- **Form**: L-carnitine comes in several forms, such as capsules, tablets, and liquids. Choose the form that best fits your preference and lifestyle.

tip n° 42
A new ally: Coenzyme Q10

Coenzyme Q10, or CoQ10, is a powerful substance that's naturally found in your body and crucial for making energy at the cellular level. Think of it as the spark that keeps the engines in your cells running, especially in energy-hungry organs like the heart, liver, and kidneys.

As we get older, our natural levels of CoQ10 can drop, which might slow our metabolism and make it harder to lose weight. Fortunately, nowadays we have the possibility of increasing your CoQ10 concentrations through supplementation. The results of recent research are optimistic and make us look at this component as a promising ally for our physical shape.

Taking CoQ10 supplements might help boost your energy production, potentially making it easier to burn fat and calories.

- **Boosts Metabolism**: CoQ10 supports the mitochondria—the powerhouses of your cells—to produce energy from nutrients. When your metabolism is running efficiently, it can help you burn calories and fat more effectively, aiding in weight loss.

- **Enhances Exercise Performance**: By boosting energy production, CoQ10 can give you the extra stamina and endurance you need for workouts. More effective workouts can lead to greater calorie burn and muscle development, both of which contribute to weight loss.

Reduces Fatigue: If you find yourself feeling tired or sluggish, CoQ10 can help combat fatigue by increasing your energy levels. This can be a game-changer for those struggling to find the motivation to exercise regularly.

Supports Heart Health: A healthy heart is crucial for effective workouts. CoQ10 has been linked to improved heart function, allowing you to engage in cardio and other intense activities without strain.

Antioxidant Properties: CoQ10 acts as an antioxidant, which can help reduce oxidative stress and inflammation in the body. Lower inflammation levels can lead to improved metabolic function, supporting your weight loss journey.

To supplement with coenzyme Q10 (CoQ10), it's generally recommended to take a daily dose between <u>30 to 200 milligrams</u>, depending on your needs and health goals.

- **Start with a Low Dose**: If you're new to CoQ10 supplements, start with a lower dose, like <u>30 to 100</u> milligrams per day. This can help you gauge how your body responds.
- **Choose the Right Form**: CoQ10 supplements come in various forms, such as softgels, capsules, and tablets. Softgels are often preferred because they're easier to swallow and can be absorbed more efficiently due to the added oils.
- **Take with Food**: CoQ10 is fat-soluble, which means it absorbs better when taken with a meal that contains some healthy fats. So, it's a good idea to take your supplement with breakfast, lunch, or dinner.

tip n° 43
Give Moro orange extract a try

Moro orange extract comes from a specific variety of blood oranges known as Moro oranges, which are primarily grown in Sicily, Italy. These oranges have a distinct deep red color inside, thanks to their high content of anthocyanins, a type of antioxidant.

Moro orange extract is made by processing these unique oranges to concentrate the beneficial compounds they contain, including the antioxidants and flavonoids. People often use this extract in dietary supplements and health products because it has benefits for weight loss and overall health.

In a simple way, you can think of Moro orange extract as a concentrated source of the good stuff found in blood oranges. It's used in supplements to support weight loss, boost metabolism, and promote a healthy immune system. Because it contains powerful natural antioxidants, it could also help combat oxidative stress and support heart health.

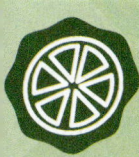

Typical Dosage: The recommended daily dosage for Moro orange extract varies, but it's generally around 400 to 800 milligrams per day. This can vary depending on the specific product and concentration of the extract, so always check the supplement label for guidance.

Supports Weight Loss: Studies suggest that Moro orange extract helps to reduce body fat by enhancing fat metabolism and reducing appetite, aiding in weight loss.

High in Antioxidants: Moro orange extract contains high levels of anthocyanins, a type of antioxidant that can help combat oxidative stress and protect cells from damage.

May Improve Metabolism: The extract has compounds that boost metabolic activity, leading to increased calorie burn and energy levels.

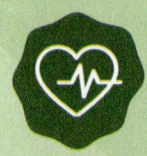

Supports Heart Health: The antioxidants and other beneficial compounds in Moro orange extract could contribute to heart health by reducing inflammation and helping to manage cholesterol levels.

May Help Control Blood Sugar: Some studies suggest that Moro orange extract could help stabilize blood sugar levels, which is important for overall health and could indirectly support weight loss.

Potential Anti-Inflammatory Properties: The extract has anti-inflammatory effects, which can be beneficial for overall well-being and reducing the risk of chronic diseases.

Here is another powerful natural extract that you can test and implement into your routine. Remember to evaluate the results and your body's response to the supplement.

tip n° 44
Don't underestimate adequate hydration

Here's a point that many people overlook while focusing on tailored meal planning for weight loss.
Studies show that dehydration or drinking insufficient water can drastically reduce metabolic reactions, in addition to signaling an increase in appetite to the brain.

Maintaining an adequate hydration pattern, especially during your weight loss and muscle gain process, is as essential as a balanced diet and exercise routine. Among the main consequences of a low level of water intake for your performance:

Slower Metabolism: When you're dehydrated, your metabolism can slow down, reducing the rate at which your body burns calories. This can make it harder to maintain a calorie deficit, which is key for weight loss.

Increased Appetite: Dehydration can cause feelings of hunger, leading to overeating or consuming unhealthy snacks. This can disrupt your weight loss efforts by causing you to consume more calories than you burn.

Reduced Energy Levels: Dehydration can make you feel tired and sluggish, which can reduce your activity levels. Lower energy can mean fewer calories burned through exercise and daily activities, making weight loss more challenging.

Increased Water Retention: Ironically, when you're dehydrated, your body may retain water as a protective mechanism, leading to bloating and weight gain. This can make it difficult to see progress on the scale, even if you're losing fat.

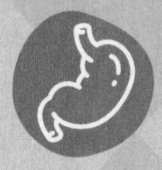

Impaired Digestion: Dehydration can affect your digestive system, leading to constipation and bloating. This can impact how your body processes food and eliminate waste, hindering weight loss.

Reduced Exercise Performance: Dehydration can impair your physical performance during workouts, reducing your ability to exercise intensely or for longer periods. This can limit calorie burn and muscle building.

Your phase of greatest physical performance must necessarily have an adequate hydration pattern. It is at this stage when you lose more liquid and need a faster and more efficient metabolism and recovery. Here is definitely a simple tip that you won't want to neglect.

Do you know how much water you need to consume daily to optimize weight loss and gain lean mass?

- **Base Level**: Start with the general recommendation of about <u>8 cups (64 ounces or 2 liters)</u> of water a day. This is a basic goal to meet your body's needs.

- **Activity Adjustment**: If you're active—like hitting the gym, going for runs, or doing any kind of exercise—you'll need more water to replace what you lose through sweat. Add at least <u>1 extra cup (8 ounces or 250 milliliters)</u> for every 30 minutes of exercise.

tip n° 45
Another interesting supplement - Psylium

Psyllium is a natural dietary fiber derived from the husks of the seeds of the Plantago ovata plant. It's commonly used as a supplement to help improve digestion and promote regularity, but it also has benefits for weight loss. When psyllium is mixed with water, it swells and forms a gel-like substance that can help you feel fuller for longer, reducing hunger and potentially lowering calorie intake.

Additionally, psyllium can reduce the caloric impact of your diet by helping to stabilize blood sugar levels, which is important for managing appetite and reducing cravings. By promoting a feeling of fullness and supporting healthy digestion, psyllium can be a helpful addition to your weight loss journey.

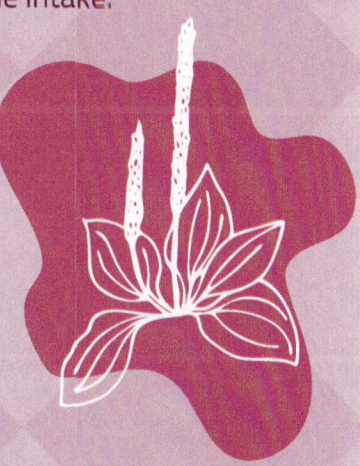

Increase Satiety: By expanding in your stomach, psyllium helps you feel fuller for a longer period. This can reduce overall calorie intake, which is helpful for weight loss.

Regulate Blood Sugar: The gel-like consistency of psyllium can slow down the absorption of sugar in your digestive system, helping to maintain stable blood sugar levels. This can prevent sudden spikes and crashes that often lead to cravings and overeating.

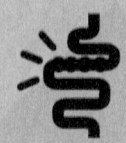

Promote Regularity: Psyllium adds bulk to stools and helps maintain regular bowel movements. This can help reduce bloating and discomfort, often associated with irregular digestion.

Lower Cholesterol: Studies suggest that psyllium can bind with cholesterol in the gut, aiding in its removal from the body. Lowering cholesterol can be beneficial for heart health, which is an important aspect of overall well-being.

Remember when we talked about the importance of adding quality fiber to your diet? Here's a great opportunity to do that while still taking advantage of Psyllium's other benefits.

- **Start with a Small Dose**: If you're new to psyllium, start with a small amount, like one teaspoon (about 5 grams) mixed with water. This helps your body adjust to the increased fiber intake.

- **Drink Plenty of Water**: Because psyllium absorbs a lot of water, it's important to stay hydrated. Drink at least 8 ounces (240 milliliters) of water with your psyllium supplement, and continue to drink water throughout the day.

- **Gradually Increase the Dose**: If you tolerate the initial dose well, you can gradually increase it to about 10-15 grams per day, spread over several servings. This could be one to two teaspoons at a time, two to three times a day.

- **When to take**: Psyllium can be taken with meals or between meals. Some people prefer taking it before meals to help curb appetite and reduce calorie intake.

tip n° 46
How to eliminate fecal matter

A considerable part of your body weight that you measure every time you weigh yourself to evaluate your results is actually water retention (which we mentioned previously) but also fecal impaction.

This happens particularly regularly when you are focused on a weight loss diet, as you consume many protein sources while trying to avoid carbohydrates.
In addition to this weight that prevents you from accurately measuring your progress in fat loss, the accumulation of fecal matter in the intestine can give the appearance of localized swelling, making your abdominal region enlarge considerably and even cause intestinal discomfort.

Fortunately, there are some natural resources to help you get rid of this accumulation of material in the intestine more easily and reduce your additional weight and waist volume in one fell swoop.

Increase Fiber Intake: Fiber helps bulk up stool and promotes regular bowel movements. Include a variety of high-fiber foods in your diet, such as whole grains, fruits, vegetables, legumes, and nuts. Aim for at least 25-30 grams of fiber per day.

Drink Plenty of Water: Staying hydrated is crucial for softening stool and facilitating its passage through the intestines. Aim to drink at least 8 glasses (64 ounces) of water per day, and more if you're active or in a hot climate.

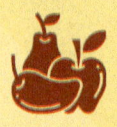

Use Natural Laxatives: Certain foods and beverages have natural laxative effects. Prunes, prune juice, and flaxseed are commonly used for this purpose. You can also try herbal teas like senna, but use them sparingly and not for long-term relief.

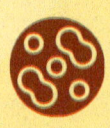

Consider Probiotics: Probiotics can help maintain a healthy gut microbiome, which is crucial for digestion and regularity. Consider adding probiotic-rich foods like yogurt, kefir, or sauerkraut to your diet, or take a high-quality probiotic supplement.

Try Glutamine: Glutamine can help with constipation by supporting intestinal health and promoting the maintenance of a healthy gut lining, which can enhance digestive function and improve bowel movements.

Quick recipe idea for constipation

Ingredients:
- 1 cup of prunes (dried plums)
- 1 tablespoon of ground flaxseed
- 1 banana
- 1 cup of almond milk
- 1 tablespoon of honey or maple
- syrup (optional)

Instructions:
- Blend the prunes, banana, and flaxseed with the almond milk until smooth.
- Add honey or maple syrup if you like it sweeter.
- Pour into a glass and enjoy!

tip n° 47

Recipe idea
Low carb dinner

Low-Carb Cauliflower Crust Pizza

Enjoy a guilt-free pizza night with this Low-Carb Cauliflower Crust Pizza. Made with a crispy cauliflower crust, topped with marinara sauce, melted mozzarella, and your favorite toppings!

Ingredients:

For the cauliflower crust:

- 1 medium head of cauliflower, riced (about 4 cups of cauliflower rice)
- 1/2 cup shredded mozzarella cheese
- 1/4 cup grated Parmesan cheese
- 1/2 teaspoon dried oregano
- 1/2 teaspoon dried basil
- 1/4 teaspoon garlic powder
- 1/4 teaspoon salt
- 1/4 teaspoon black pepper
- 1 egg

For the toppings:

- 1/2 cup sugar-free marinara sauce
- 1 cup shredded mozzarella cheese
- Your choice of toppings

Instructions:

Preheat the oven: Preheat your oven to 425°F (220°C). Line a baking sheet with parchment paper and set aside.

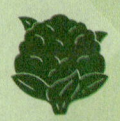

Prepare the cauliflower rice: Cut the cauliflower into florets and pulse them in a food processor until they resemble rice grains. Alternatively, you can grate the cauliflower using a box grater. You should have about 4 cups of cauliflower rice.

Cook the cauliflower rice: Place the cauliflower rice in a microwave-safe bowl and microwave on high for 5-6 minutes, or until the cauliflower is soft and tender. Allow it to cool for a few minutes.

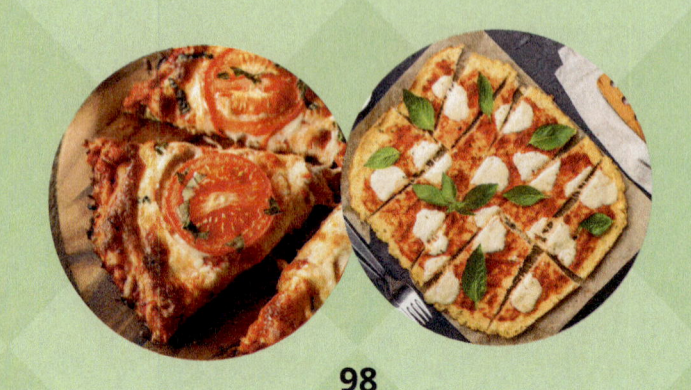

Make the cauliflower crust: Once the cauliflower has cooled, place it in a clean kitchen towel or cheesecloth and squeeze out as much moisture as possible. Transfer the squeezed cauliflower to a mixing bowl. Add shredded mozzarella cheese, grated Parmesan cheese, dried oregano, dried basil, garlic powder, salt, pepper, and the egg.
Mix until everything is well combined.

Form the crust: Transfer the cauliflower mixture to the prepared baking sheet lined with parchment paper. Use your hands to press the mixture into a thin, even circle, about 1/4 inch thick, forming a crust shape.

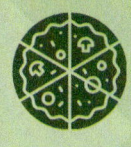

Bake the crust: Place the cauliflower crust in the preheated oven and bake for 20-25 minutes, or until the edges are golden brown and the crust is firm.

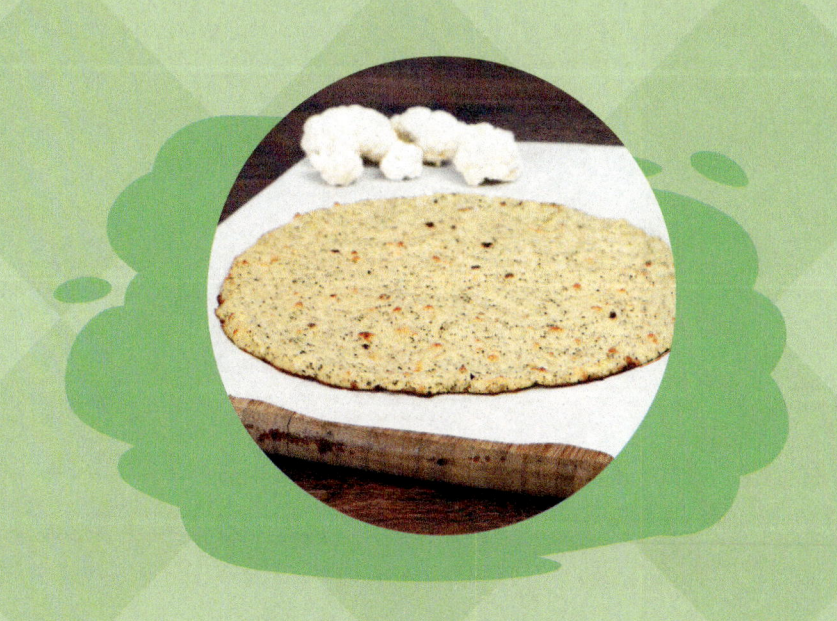

Add toppings: Once the crust is baked, remove it from the oven and spread the sugar-free marinara sauce evenly over the crust, leaving a small border around the edges. Sprinkle shredded mozzarella cheese on top of the sauce, then add your desired toppings.

Bake again: Return the pizza to the oven and bake for an additional 10-12 minutes, or until the cheese is melted and bubbly.

Serve: Once the pizza is cooked to your liking, remove it from the oven and let it cool for a few minutes before slicing. Serve your low-carb cauliflower crust pizza hot and enjoy!

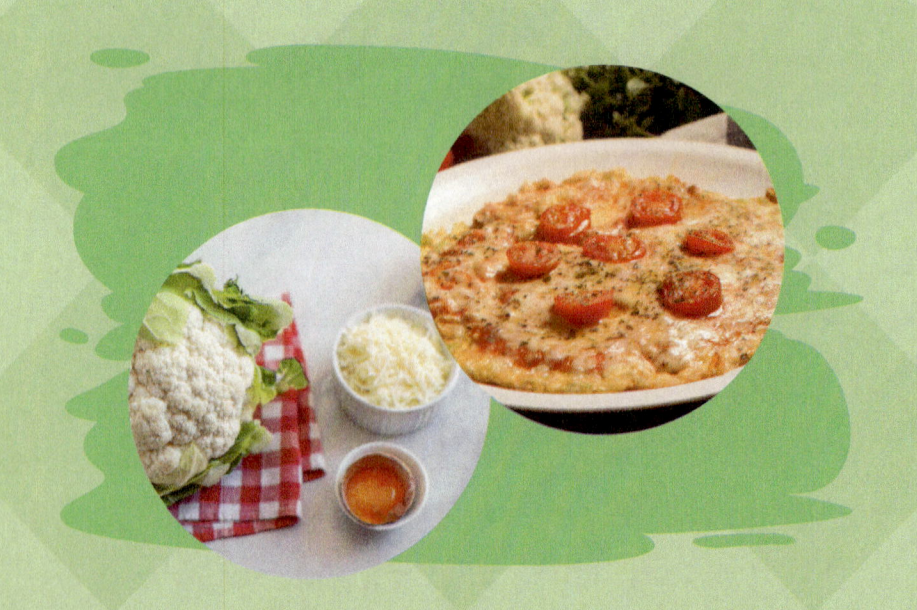

tip n° 48
Pay attention to Selenium deficiency

Selenium, a trace mineral found in various foods and essential for good health, plays a crucial role in metabolism, thyroid function, and even muscle growth. If you're trying to lose weight or gain muscle, selenium deficiency could be a hidden obstacle in your journey. This mineral is key to regulating thyroid hormones, which are involved in controlling your body's metabolism. Without enough selenium, you might experience slower metabolism, fatigue, and even muscle weakness, all of which can hinder your weight loss and muscle gain goals. In this chapter, we'll explore the importance of selenium, how to identify a deficiency, and ways to ensure you're getting enough to support your fitness journey. Let's dive in!

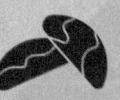

Brazil Nuts: These are one of the richest sources of selenium, with just one or two nuts providing the recommended daily intake.

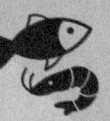

Seafood: Fish and shellfish, such as tuna, sardines, halibut, shrimp, and salmon, contain high levels of selenium.

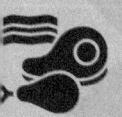

Meat: Poultry, beef, pork, and lamb are also good sources of selenium.

Eggs: Eggs contain a moderate amount of selenium, making them a convenient source of the mineral.

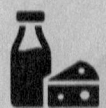

Dairy Products: Milk, cheese, and yogurt contain selenium, though in smaller amounts compared to seafood and meats.

Whole Grains: Foods like whole wheat bread, brown rice, and oatmeal can provide a modest amount of selenium.

Sunflower Seeds: These seeds offer a decent amount of selenium and can be a great addition to snacks or salads.

Including a variety of these selenium-rich foods in your diet can help ensure you're getting enough of this important mineral to support your overall health, including metabolism, thyroid function, and muscle growth.

However, if you suspect that you are consuming a low dosage of Selenium daily, you may be inclined to supplement with the mineral following a recommended daily dosage:

Start with the Recommended Daily Intake: For most adults, the recommended daily intake of selenium is about 55 micrograms (mcg).

Take with Food: Selenium supplements are generally best taken with food. This helps with absorption and can reduce the chance of an upset stomach. Try to take it with a meal or a snack to get the most benefit.

tip n° 49
Also bet on Glucomannan

If you are willing and motivated to start a journey to lose fat, but one of your biggest concerns is binge eating and lack of discipline to maintain a healthy eating habit, pay attention to this next tip. This is another powerful compound proven to be efficient in controlling and reducing appetite, and can become one of your best allies.

Glucomannan is a unique, water-soluble dietary fiber derived from the root of the konjac plant (Amorphophallus konjac), native to Southeast Asia. It is known for its ability to absorb water and expand in the stomach, which can help with weight loss by promoting feelings of fullness and reducing overall calorie intake. This effect can lead to reduced snacking and smaller portion sizes, supporting weight loss.

Scientifically, glucomannan has been shown to slow the absorption of glucose and dietary fat, which can help maintain steady blood sugar levels and support heart health. Additionally, by adding bulk to the stool, it may improve bowel regularity and aid digestion.

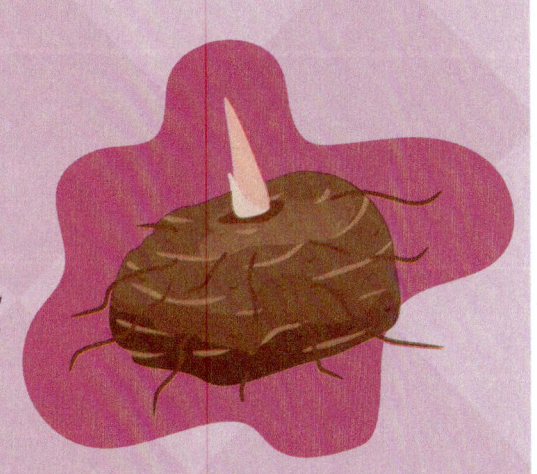

Several studies have indicated that glucomannan supplementation can contribute to weight loss when combined with a calorie-controlled diet and exercise. However, it's crucial to use it as directed, with plenty of water, to avoid potential issues like choking or blockages, given its strong water-absorbing properties. As with any supplement, consult a healthcare provider before use, especially if you have existing medical conditions or are on medication.

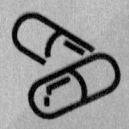

Start Small: If you're new to glucomannan, start with a smaller dose to see how your body reacts. A common starting point is 500 mg, taken once a day.

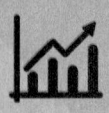

Increase Gradually: Once you've established your tolerance, you can increase your dose. The typical recommended dose is 1 to 2 grams, taken three times a day, but always follow the product's instructions or your healthcare provider's advice.

Take with Water: Glucomannan needs plenty of water to work properly. Always take it with at least 8 ounces of water. This helps it expand and prevents the risk of choking or blockages in your throat or digestive tract.

Timing Is Key: For weight loss, the best time to take glucomannan is about 15 to 30 minutes before meals. This allows it to expand in your stomach, helping you feel fuller and eat smaller portions during your meal.

tip nº 50
Pure strength workouts

Many times during your journey of physical evolution, you may not be achieving satisfactory results as before because you do not have enough brute strength to progress the weights and continue giving considerable stimulation to your muscles.

Progressing your strength and muscle pulling capacity can be a game changer for you. If this is the variable that is preventing you from evolving further, applying these tips will certainly bring quick results. Brute strength is essential both to progress in gaining muscle mass and to ensure sufficient muscle stimulation during fat loss, and to avoid "catalysis" or loss of lean mass in this process, preserving your muscle mass while you only lose fat.

Muscle fibers are the cells or basic building blocks of muscle tissue, and they play a crucial role in determining how strong and powerful you can be. When we talk about brute strength, we're generally referring to the ability to generate a lot of force, often in a short amount of time. This ability largely depends on a specific type of muscle fiber known as "fast-twitch" fibers.

Fast-Twitch Muscle Fibers: These fibers are built for fast, explosive movements and are vital for generating high force, making them essential for brute strength activities like heavy weightlifting, powerlifting, and sprinting. Although they have less endurance than "slow-twitch" fibers, they produce more power in a shorter time.

Adapted training to increase strength:

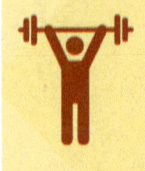

Choose Compound Exercises: Focus on compound exercises that work multiple muscle groups at once. This approach not only saves time but also encourages overall muscle growth and strength. Key compound exercises include squats, deadlifts, bench presses, shoulder presses, and pull-ups.

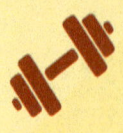

Use Heavy Weights with Low Repetitions: For strength training, you want to lift heavy weights with lower repetitions. Aim for <u>4 to 6 repetitions</u> per set, with a weight that's challenging but allows you to maintain good form. This range is optimal for building brute strength.

Rest Between Sets: When training for strength, it's important to give your muscles time to recover between sets. Rest for about <u>2 to 3 minutes</u> before moving on to the next set. This rest period allows your muscles to recover enough to lift heavy weights again.

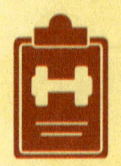

Follow a Structured Program: Consistency is key, so follow a structured training program. A common approach is to work different muscle groups on specific days. For example:
- Day 1: Upper body (bench press, shoulder press, rows)
- Day 2: Lower body (squats, deadlifts, lunges)
- Day 3: Rest or light activity
- Day 4: Upper body (pull-ups, dips, incline bench press)
- Day 5: Lower body (leg press, Romanian deadlift, calf raises)
- Day 6 and 7: Rest or light activity

tip n° 51
Combine strategies intelligently

Firstly, congratulations on getting this far. The vast majority of people who seek changes in all areas of life generally do not achieve satisfactory results simply because they are too lazy to take the time to learn and study the mechanism of things first.

Now that you've come this far, you have at your disposal a wide range of practical and scientifically validated information about weight loss and muscle mass gain and you are a big step ahead of most people.

The idea here is not to try to apply all these tips simultaneously, but rather to use this valuable knowledge gradually throughout your process each time results stagnate.

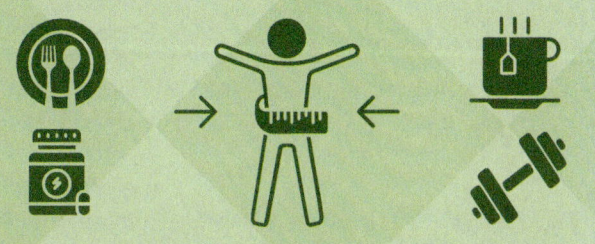

Now you know different advanced strategies, and you can make small adjustments to your routine, implementing these tips in whatever way is most convenient and comfortable for you and your lifestyle.

Apply some of these diet tips in conjunction with some advanced strategies focused on physical activity and, when you deem it necessary, add a new variable or stimulus such as extracts, teas, supplements, or alternative strategies.

Imagine you're on a journey to a healthier you, and you're making great progress. But suddenly, it feels like you've hit a roadblock — you're not losing weight anymore, no matter how hard you try.

You have reached a plateau! And that is exactly why most people are unable to achieve satisfactory results, much less maintain them.

That's where breaking plateau strategies come in! Over time you will need more advanced strategies and stronger stimuli to continue progressing. You will aways have an ace up your sleeve!

Use the scale to evaluate your results, but also get into the habit of looking in the mirror regularly, as you can gain a little weight due to muscle mass gain, fecal cake or water retention too.

Now you are equipped with the best alternatives to continue improving your evolutionary process.
Be persistent but patient. Every process of drastic change in our physique is essentially a medium and long-term project. But make sure you are evolving a little every day.

Printed in Great Britain
by Amazon